Reading Success in the Primary Years

Marleen F. Westerveld · Rebecca M. Armstrong ·
Georgina M. Barton

Reading Success in the Primary Years

An Evidence-Based Interdisciplinary Approach to Guide Assessment and Intervention

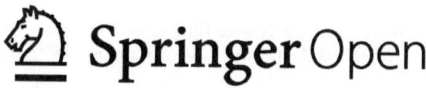

Marleen F. Westerveld
Griffith University
Southport, QLD, Australia

Rebecca M. Armstrong
University of Queensland
St Lucia, QLD, Australia

Georgina M. Barton
University of Southern Queensland
Springfield Central, QLD, Australia

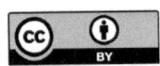

ISBN 978-981-15-3491-1   ISBN 978-981-15-3492-8   (eBook)
https://doi.org/10.1007/978-981-15-3492-8

This Springer imprint is published by the registered company Springer Nature Singapore Pte Ltd.
The registered company address is: 152 Beach Road, #21-01/04 Gateway East, Singapore 189721,
Singapore

Preface

The overall aim of the *Reading Success* project described in this book is the systematic and accurate identification of students' reading profiles within a primary school setting in Australia to better support the reading outcomes of those students who struggle in reading. We embraced an education–speech pathology collaborative practice model (see Archibald, 2017), in line with speech pathology Australia's clinical guideline for speech pathologists working in literacy (Serry et al., 2016). In this study, we adopted a range of evidence-based frameworks and approaches, including the Simple View of Reading (Gough & Tunmer, 1986), and a response-to-intervention approach (Jimerson, Burns, & van der Heyden, 2015). The study involved a strong partnership between all stakeholders including academic researchers in speech pathology and education and research end-users at the school.

In an attempt to bridge the research-to-practice gap, we present a five-step assessment to intervention process involved in implementing an interdisciplinary and evidence-based approach to the identification of and support for students at risk for or experiencing difficulties in reading in a school setting. We share participants' perspectives, gathered throughout the study, including the views from leaders, teachers, students, and support staff, such as speech pathologists within the school context. As our aim in this project was not to describe or evaluate current literacy practices, we did not systematically gather information on classroom literacy practices. However, we provide an easily accessible overview of a range of evidence-based and theoretically driven initiatives aimed at enhancing the reading success of primary (or elementary)-aged students in schools. Upon implementing our five-step assessment to intervention framework, schools will be able to (i) identify which students are in need of extra support to facilitate reading success; (ii) create individual speech-to-print profiles for students who show difficulties in reading comprehension; and (iii) initiate targeted support for students with reading difficulties that is firmly based on the assessment results (Munro, 2017).

Throughout the book, there is a clear focus on how the team worked collaboratively across different year levels, which included the decision-making processes used, such as rich dialogue with the leadership team and teachers. As such, it offers valuable insights for educators, speech pathologists, researchers, and pre-service teacher education students interested in promoting reading success within a school setting. We discuss these implications and future directions in more detail in the final chapter of this book.

Southport, Australia   Marleen F. Westerveld
St Lucia, Australia   Rebecca M. Armstrong
Springfield Central, Australia   Georgina M. Barton

References

Archibald, L. M. (2017). SLP-educator classroom collaboration: A review to inform reason-based practice. *Autism & Developmental Language Impairments*, *2*, 1–17. https://doi.org/10.1177/2396941516680369.

Gough, P. B., & Tunmer, W. E. (1986). Decoding, reading, and reading disability. *Remedial and Special Education*, *7*(1), 6–10. https://doi.org/10.1177/074193258600700104.

Jimerson, S. R., Burns, M. K., & VanDerHeyden, A. M. (Eds.). (2015). *Handbook of response to intervention: The science and practice of multi-tiered systems of support* (2nd ed.). New York: Springer.

Munro, J. (2017). Who benefits from which reading intervention in the primary years? Match the intervention with the reading profile. *Australian Journal of Learning Difficulties*, *22*(2), 133–151. https://doi.org/10.1080/19404158.2017.1379027.

Serry, T., Jones, E., Walmsley, K., Westerveld, M. F., Neilson, R., Leitao, S., & Rowe, T. (2016). Clinical guidelines for speech pathologists working in literacy. Melbourne, Victoria: Speech Pathology Australia.

Acknowledgements

We would like to acknowledge everyone involved in the Reading Success project. First and foremost, we would like to thank the teachers and leadership team at the school for their willingness to share their time, expertise, and passion for the teaching of reading. Without their firm, enduring support and enthusiasm, this project would not have been possible. We would also like to thank the families and children involved in the project, for allowing us to conduct the assessments and follow the children's progress in reading over a couple of years. The project would not have been possible without the amazing speech pathologists Bronte Brook, Kate O'Leary, Caitlin O'Rourke, and Susan Collecutt; your commitment to the project has been outstanding.

We would also like to acknowledge our co-authors for sharing their expertise and perspectives. We have learnt so much from this interdisciplinary collaboration and hope this is reflected in the text. While we acknowledge there are different opinions and philosophies towards the teaching of reading, at the core of this study was a shared vision to support students in becoming successful readers. Finally, a big thank you to some wonderful colleagues for proofreading the book and providing us with constructive feedback. You know who you are!

This project was supported, in kind, by the Department of Education; the views expressed in this publication are not necessarily the views of the department.

Contents

8 Implications and Transferability to Other School Contexts 141

Marleen F. Westerveld, Rebecca M. Armstrong, Georgina M. Barton,
and Jennifer Peach

Authors and Contributor

About the Authors

Marleen F. Westerveld, Ph.D. is an Associate Professor in speech pathology in the School of Allied Health Sciences at Griffith University and a Member of the Menzies Health Institute Queensland, Australia. She has a solid track record in applied research in the areas of (emergent) literacy and oral language development in typically developing children, children with developmental language disorders, and children with language disorders associated with biomedical conditions, such as Down syndrome and autism spectrum disorder. She is the principal investigator on numerous funded research projects aimed (directly or indirectly) at improving the spoken and/or written communication skills of children, adolescents, and young adults. Her work has resulted in more than 60 published research papers in high-quality peer-reviewed national and international journals on topics of language and literacy. She is currently Editor for Language, Speech, and Hearing Services in Schools and Chair of the Child Language Committee of the International Association of Logopedics and Phoniatrics.
 e-mail: m.westerveld@griffith.edu.au

Rebecca M. Armstrong, Ph.D. is a Lecturer in speech pathology at the University of Queensland in Australia. She has worked clinically as Speech Pathologist in the Department of Education (Queensland) prior to commencing her academic appointment at the University of Queensland. In the higher education sector, she teaches across the undergraduate and master's speech pathology programmes in a range of paediatric areas. She researches in the areas of language and literacy for school-aged populations, including children with autism spectrum disorders. She also has a research track record in population-based research examining the early life predictors and long-term outcomes of language impairment.
 e-mail: rebecca.armstrong@uq.edu.au

Georgina M. Barton, Ph.D. is a Professor in the School of Education at the University of Southern Queensland in Australia where she is Associate Head of School (research) and Discipline Lead for literacy and pedagogy. She has taught in a number of schools and has experience as Acting Principal and working as a volunteer in South India teaching English. In the higher education context, she has taught English and literacy, and arts education. She researches in the areas of the arts and literacy with diverse communities and has attracted over $1.4 million in research funding as both Project Leader and Member of teams. With over 120 publications, she has utilised a range of methodologies including arts-based research, case study design, ethnography, and narrative inquiry. Her latest book is *Developing Literacy and the Arts in Schools* with Routledge Publishers. e-mail: georgina.barton@usq.edu.au

Contributor

Jennifer Peach is a certified practising Speech Pathologist with extensive experience in the application of speech pathology in an educational context. In her current role as Senior Advisor in speech-language therapy at the Queensland Department of Education's Reading Centre, she provides professional leadership and learning opportunities to build system and educator capability to identify students experiencing difficulties learning to read, and to provide the necessary adjustments and supports for students with reading disorders to access age-appropriate curriculum. e-mail: Jennifer.PEACH@qed.qld.gov.au

Chapter 1
Reading Success

Marleen F. Westerveld, Rebecca M. Armstrong, and Georgina M. Barton

Abstract This chapter explains what skills are needed for reading success. It highlights the Simple View of Reading and its core components, word recognition and language comprehension, and how it may be used as a guiding framework across different year levels to describe students' reading abilities and/or difficulties, plan subsequent intervention, and monitor progress. We describe the underlying spoken and written language skills needed for successful reading comprehension including both cognitive and sociocultural approaches to making meaning. We share how creating speech-to-print profiles for those students who need further support in reading comprehension may inform instructional practice, using a multi-tiered system of support approach. The importance of an evidence-based, collaborative, interdisciplinary approach to identying and supporting students experiencing difficulties in reading is highlighted. Finally, an explanation of the importance of providing research-based reading supports at increasingly intense levels matched to the student's needs is provided.

Keywords Simple view of reading · Reading comprehension · Speech-to-print profile

1.1 Introduction

In response to the comparatively low levels of reading performance of Australian primary school students compared to international benchmarks (Mullis, Martin, Foy, & Drucker, 2012), the teaching of reading in Australian classrooms has received considerable attention by a diverse group of stakeholders, including policy-makers (Australian Government, 2005, 2015) and education professionals (Stark, Snow, Eadie, & Goldfeld, 2016). As outlined in an influential Australian Government report, the Teacher Education Ministerial Advisory Group (TEMAG) (Australian Government, 2015), there is a critical need to lift student outcomes. This scene is similar in many other countries and reflects other reports such as the No Child Left Behind Act (2002) and the National Reading Panel (2000) in the USA. As such, this book shares findings from a research project, aimed to improve reading outcomes, implemented in one school in Queensland, Australia.

© The Author(s) 2020
M. F. Westerveld et al., *Reading Success in the Primary Years*,
https://doi.org/10.1007/978-981-15-3492-8_1

1

Reading is a complex human behaviour. The ultimate goal of all reading is reading comprehension, the ability to gain meaning from text. The importance of successful reading comprehension for academic success, socio-emotional well-being, and employment outcomes is undisputable (McGeown, Duncan, Griffiths, & Stothard, 2015), and it is therefore no surprise that a wealth of research exists investigating not only how students acquire and develop their reading skills, but also what successful intervention looks like when students struggle in their reading development (e.g. Amendum, Bratsch-Hines, & Vernon-Feagans, 2018; Clarke, Snowling, Truelove, & Hulme, 2010; Snowling & Hulme, 2011). Unfortunately, a research-to-practice gap still exists, with many professionals involved in the teaching of reading unsure how to bridge that gap. We agree with Tunmer and Hoover (2019) that a clearly defined theoretical framework that underpins assessment and intervention will assist reading professionals in developing the competencies needed to better understand why some children struggle with reading and how to provide targeted support and intervention. This chapter therefore starts by introducing some theoretical frameworks to better understand what is involved in successful reading comprehension.

1.2   Theoretical Frameworks

1.2.1   The Construction-Integration Model

According to the construction-integration model put forward by Kintsch (1988), successful text comprehension (albeit spoken or written) relies on the interaction between bottom-up and top-down processes at three levels: the surface level, the propositional level, and the situation level. The reader must first read and attach a linguistic representation to the word/s on a page (literal or surface representations). By connecting these words or propositions and through making inferences, the reader then forms an overall representation of the meaning of what was read (the propositional level or the text base). Finally, a situation (or mental) model is formed by activating *background knowledge* and *schemas* related to the text *in long-term memory*. A study by Oakhill and Cain (2012) demonstrated that the ability to construct a "coherent and integrated representation of the meaning of a text" (p. 116) predicts reading comprehension. More specifically, when investigating the predictors of reading comprehension in 83 children attending Year 6 (ages 10–11), based on their performance in Year 3 (ages 7–8) and Year 4 (ages 8–9), Oakhill and Cain found that Year 4 inferencing, Year 4 comprehension monitoring, and Year 3 knowledge and use of text structure were distinct predictors of reading comprehension in Year 6. This occurred even after controlling for reading comprehension ability at Year 3 and accounting for vocabulary knowledge and verbal IQ. We will discuss some of these concepts in more detail.

Inferencing. Inferencing or the ability to go beyond what is explicitly stated by making links between words or sentences plays an important role in the reading comprehension process, both concurrently and longitudinally. Oakhill and Cain (2012) investigated the predictors of reading comprehension in 102 children between ages 7 and 8 (Year 3 of schooling) and 10–11 (Year 6) and found inferencing to be one of three distinct predictors of reading comprehension in Year 6, once reading comprehension ability at Year 3, vocabulary knowledge, and IQ were accounted for. Inferential comprehension generally develops from an early age and includes drawing links to fill gaps in the information provided, drawing meaning from prior knowledge, linking relations between information, and forming predictions. For example, consider the sentence 'Rosie went outside and took an umbrella'. To understand this sentence, the reader must draw on prior knowledge to understand that we generally use umbrellas to shield us from the rain.

Comprehension monitoring. Another distinct predictor of reading comprehension in Year 6 is comprehension monitoring, which refers to the child's ability to reflect on what has just been read and to look for inconsistencies in a text. Students with poor comprehension often focus more on word accuracy than comprehension monitoring and generally have weaker metacognition skills (Nation & Norbury, 2005). Although it is difficult to disentangle the causal relationship between inferencing ability and comprehension monitoring, it has been well established that children who demonstrate reading comprehension difficulties often perform poorly on tasks measuring comprehension monitoring (Oakhill, Hartt, & Samols, 2005).

Text structure knowledge. Text structure knowledge refers to the readers' knowledge of the typical structure of a text. One well-known example of a text structure associated with narratives is story grammar (Stein & Glenn, 1979). Most narratives (or stories) are goal-oriented and contain the following elements of setting, characters, problem, plan, actions, resolution, and conclusion. This text structure knowledge may assist comprehension by allowing the reader to link the ideas presented in the story and by creating expectations of what may happen next. It is thus not surprising that knowledge of text structure assists in reading comprehension. Research has clearly demonstrated that students with poor reading comprehension often struggle in their ability to tell well-structured narratives (e.g. Westerveld, Gillon, & Moran, 2008) and that poor story structure knowledge may in fact cause some of these readers' comprehension difficulties (Cain & Oakhill, 1996).

1.2.2 The Simple View of Reading

A theoretical framework that has received much attention in the last 30 years is the Simple View of Reading (SVR) (Gough & Tunmer, 1986). Unlike the construction-integration model (Kintsch, 1988), it does not attempt to explain the cognitive underpinnings of the reading process, but it outlines which core components are involved in reading comprehension. The SVR holds that reading comprehension is the product of word recognition and language comprehension. The significant aspect of the SVR is that reading is conceptualised as a product of both components rather than an accrual. If one component is poor or non-existent, reading comprehension competency will not be fully achieved. *Word recognition* (WR) can be defined as the ability to accurately and efficiently decode the written words on a page, whereas *language comprehension* (LC) involves the understanding of spoken language at word (vocabulary), sentence (syntax), and text (e.g. narrative) levels (Catts, Adlof, & Ellis Weismer, 2006). More recently, an update to the SVR has been published by Tunmer and Hoover (2019), referred to as the Cognitive Foundations Framework. This framework more clearly explains the cognitive 'capacities' needed for language comprehension, namely (a) linguistic knowledge, including phonological knowledge, semantic knowledge, and syntactic knowledge needed for literal interpretation of language, and (b) background knowledge and inferencing skills, which are often influenced by sociocultural aspects of children's lives. A combination of all these knowledge constructs and skills will assist the reader or listener to understand and use language effectively.

The SVR has received considerable attention in the research literature, and while there is some controversy surrounding this perspective, results have shown that the two components (WR and LC) account for almost all of the variance in reading comprehension in students learning English as a first language/writing system (Catts, Hogan, & Adlof, 2005; Lonigan, Burgess, & Schatschneider, 2018), as well as those students who are learning English as a second language (e.g. Verhoeven & van Leeuwe, 2012). It should be noted, however, that the relative and unique contributions of WR and LC to RC change over time. During the early stages of *learning to read*, typically during the first three years of schooling, WR shows the biggest contribution to RC. This is not surprising as almost all children come to reading instruction with better oral language skills than decoding skills and as such early reading materials will often not challenge a student's language comprehension. Once students have learned to master fluent and accurate word reading, usually around their fourth year of schooling, and make the transition from learning to read to *reading to learn*, LC demonstrates the biggest contribution to RC (Catts, Hogan, & Adlof, 2005). At this stage of the reading process, reading materials have become more linguistically challenging, with more abstract words, more complex grammar, and more advanced text structures. Although there is clear evidence of the unique contributions of WR and LC to RC, up to 69% of the variance accounted for in RC points to shared contribution of word recognition and language comprehension. For example, a student's ability to efficiently recognise a real word (as opposed to a nonsense word) may be facilitated by this same student's vocabulary knowledge (which is an aspect of language comprehension). These results indicate that for students who fail to show adequate progress in reading comprehension, intervention may need to target both LC and WR.

1.3   Emergent Literacy Skills

Children's literacy learning starts at birth, long before children commence their formal reading education at school. During this period, also referred to as the emergent literacy stage (Justice, 2006), children are typically engaged in a range of literacy-related activities, such as : (a) shared book reading with their parents or early childhood educators; (b) exposure to environmental print (e.g. *M* for McDonalds); (c) access to writing utensils to 'write' their name; and (d) other literate practices appropriate for their sociocultural surroundings such as oral storytelling. The development of emergent literacy skills may be influenced by environmental factors such as family trauma, displacement, and/or economic hardship or affluence. Regardless, research demonstrates that the following five emergent literacy skills are strongly predictive of future reading success (National Early Literacy Panel, 2008), even after controlling for socio-economic status and cognition (IQ): alphabet knowledge, phonological awareness, rapid automatic naming of (a) digits and (b) objects, emergent name writing, and phonological memory. Five additional skills were identified that showed strong correlations but needed some further research, including print concepts and oral language (vocabulary and grammar). Table 1.1 provides an overview of this terminology. Using the SVR as a framework, these emergent literacy skills may be conceptualised as the code-related skills that are needed for future word recognition and the meaning-related skills required for successful language comprehension (NICHD, 2005).

1.4 Classifying Struggling Readers

Using the SVR as a theoretical framework, students who are unable to develop adequate reading comprehension skills can be categorised into three main groups: (1) students with dyslexia are those who show significant word reading difficulties, in the absence of language comprehension problems; (2) students with specific comprehension difficulties are those who show adequate word recognition skills, but significant language comprehension difficulties; (3) students with a mixed reading difficulties profile (in the past referred to as garden variety poor readers) are those who show weaknesses across word recognition and language comprehension (Spear-Swerling, 2016). These three reader groups are discussed in a little more detail below:

Dyslexia or Specific Word Reading Difficulties These reading difficulties stem from phonological processing weaknesses (including phonological awareness, rapid automatic naming [RAN], and/or phonological memory). Students who show this reading profile have adequate vocabulary and language comprehension skills. These students will demonstrate reading comprehension difficulties due to their weaknesses in accurate and/or fluent word recognition skills. It is estimated that approximately 5–10% of students will show dyslexia (Catts, Hogan, & Adlof, 2005; Shaywitz, Shaywitz, Fletcher, & Escobar, 1990).

Specific Comprehension Difficulties These students will demonstrate reading comprehension difficulties, despite adequate word recognition skills (accuracy and fluency). These students will often demonstrate language comprehension weaknesses across vocabulary, grammar, and oral narrative/higher-order language skills (Catts et al., 2006; Woolley, 2011). In addition, these students may lack a strategic approach to comprehension of text (Spear-Swerling, 2015). Research has shown that up to 17% of students may show this type of reading difficulty.

Table 1.1 Overview of (emergent) literacy skills with definitions (NELP, 2008) and examples of assessment tasks

Code-related emergent literacy skills	The skills that are strongly predictive of word recognition.	Examples of assessment tasks
Phonological awareness	The child's ability to consciously identify sounds in spoken language, including syllables, onset-rime, and individual sounds (phonemes). Note: phonemic awareness refers to this awareness at the phoneme (sound) level only.	Syllables: How many syllables/claps in elephant? Answer: 3: e/le/phant. Onset-rime: what is the first sound in bed? Answer: /b/ Phonemes: how many sounds in bed? Answer: 3: /b/ /e/ /d/
Alphabet knowledge (phonics)	The child's ability to name and/or provide the sounds of printed letters, including *Single letters, Digraphs, Diphthongs Trigraphs*	Single letters: all 26 letters of the alphabet. Digraphs: /sh/ /th/ /kn/ etc Diphthongs: /oi/ /oo/ /ow/ etc Trigraphs: /igh/ /tch/ etc
Emergent (name) writing	The child's ability to write letters when requested and/or to write his/her own name	Provide the child with a blank piece of paper and a pen/pencil: Can you write your name?
Rapid automatic naming (RAN) of letters/digits	The child's ability to rapidly name a sequence of letters/digits	The child is provided with a sheet of paper containing familiar pictures, digits, or coloured shapes and asked to name as many as they can in 60 seconds.
Rapid automatic naming (RAN) of objects or colours	The child's ability to rapidly name sets of pictures or colours	
Phonological memory	The child's ability to remember verbal information for a short period of time	For example, ask the child to repeat non-words: *flibvat*, or *striken*
Print concepts	The child's knowledge of print conventions	For example, reading from left to right and understanding that written text carries meaning.
Meaning-related emergent literacy skills	The skills that are strongly predictive of language comprehension	
Vocabulary	The child's knowledge of spoken words	The child is asked to point to a picture (choice of four) in response to a spoken word.
Grammar	The child's knowledge of the rules of the English language.	The child is asked to point to a picture (choice of four) in response to a short sentence e.g. *The star is in the ball.*
Narrative skills	The child's ability to comprehend and re/tell a coherent well-sequenced story.	The child is asked several questions after listening to a novel story. The child is then asked to re/tell the story.

Mixed Reading Difficulties These students show a combination of word recognition and language comprehension weaknesses (as per the preceding two profiles). It is estimated that approximately 30% of all students who struggle in their reading comprehension skill will have this type of reading profile.

Unfortunately, as with any theoretical model, in practice, when applying the SVR framework approximately 7.5% of children may present with 'unexplained' or 'non-specified' reading comprehension problems as their performance on the RC assessment can not be explained by challenges in their language comprehension or reading accuracy (Catts, Hogan, & Fey, 2003). Although further research will be needed to better understand why this subgroup of children have difficulties in reading comprehension, as we describe a little later in this chapter, it could be that other sociocultural factors influence their participation and therefore achievement level, for example, childhood trauma (Thompson & Whimper, 2010). Other likely explanations include the child's world knowledge, the child's motivation or understanding about the purpose of reading, as well as important executive functioning skills including sustained attention and working memory. For example, according to a limited capacity working memory model (Crystal, 1987), students who use up most of their cognitive resources for decoding (e.g. those who have not yet developed automaticity in word recognition and may resort to sounding out individual words) may have few cognitive resources available for reading comprehension. Regardless, distinguishing between these reading groups is important, as "differentiating classroom instruction according to different patterns […] may improve reading outcomes" (Spear-Swerling, 2016, p. 514).

1.5 Reading Comprehension is a Complex Process

The main focus of this book is on the cognitive skills underpinning reading development, but we recognise that other factors play an important role in the student's reading development, such as sociocultural environment (Marjanovič-Umek, Fekonja-Peklaj, Sočan, & Tašner, 2015). Although the SVR has been well-validated, reading comprehension itself is a complex multidimensional process (Catts, 2018). Further, Snow (2002) states that:

> reading comprehension is the process of simultaneously extracting and constructing meaning through interaction and involvement with written language. We use the words extracting and constructing to emphasize both the importance and the insufficiency of the text as a determinant of reading comprehension. Comprehension entails three elements:• The reader who is doing the comprehending • The text that is to be comprehended • The activity in which comprehension is a part. (p. 11)

When investigating reading comprehension, we thus need to consider what the reader brings to the process, including the reader's reading experience, world knowledge, motivation, and self-perception, as well as their overall cognitive and linguistic (oral language) skills. We acknowledge the need to take a holistic approach and include consideration of the purpose of reading and the type of texts students engage with.

Consequently, we aim to present a broad view of the 'teaching of reading' by focusing on the identification of and support for students who may be experiencing difficulties learning to read. At the same time we acknowledge this book presents an approach adopted for the purpose of our study that may be transferable to other contexts (see Chap. 8).

1.5.1   Motivation and Self-perception

Although not the main focus in this book, the importance of reading motivation and self-concept cannot be underestimated. Motivation for reading develops early in life when children start building their emergent literacy skills. As outlined by Katzir, Lesaux, and Kim (2009), research has shown that parents' identification of pleasure as a reason for reading predicted motivation for reading in their young school-aged children. Moreover, early success or difficulties in learning to read is linked to reading self-concept and motivation. In other words, if children perceive to perform well, i.e. experience success in reading, they will be motivated to challenge themselves and attempt more difficult tasks. On the other hand, if children have challenges in learning to read, their reading self-concept may weaken and these children may lose motivation in reading-related tasks. Chapman and Tunmer (1995) conceptualised reading concept as comprising three components: perceptions of competence, perceptions of difficulty or ease of reading tasks, and attitudes towards reading, and developed the *Reading Self-Concept Scale* (RSCS). Researchers applying this scale found reading self-concept positively relate to reading comprehension in primary school-aged students (Chapman & Tunmer, 1995; see also Chapman & Tunmer, 2003), even after controlling for the children's verbal ability (based on a verbal IQ test) and their word reading ability (Katzir et al., 2009). In the Reading Success project, we measured students' reading self-concept using the RSCS and report the results in Chap. 4.

1.5.2   Reading for Pleasure

It would be remiss not to mention reading for pleasure (Cremin, Mottram, Collins, Powell, & Safford, 2014). Students need to be given the time to make choices about what they read and particularly in areas of personal interest. It is important not only that children are aware of the benefit of learning to read in relation to academic success but that reading can be a 'delightful' and 'desirable' endeavour (Cremin, 2007). Much research points to the importance of developing positive classroom environments with effective communities of readers (Cremin et al., 2014) that encourage imaginative thought and playfulness. Further, the social aspect of reading, when supported, results in stronger engagement and consequently high achievement across all aspects of schooling (Ivey, 2014).

1.6 Teaching Reading During the Early Years of Schooling

1.6.1 Systematic and Explicit Teaching of the Key Ingredients

There is clear evidence that the best way to teach children how to effectively learn to read is by explicitly teaching the following five key ingredients: (1) phonics; (2) phonemic awareness; (3) fluency (the ability to recognise words automatically); (4) vocabulary; and (5) comprehension (i.e. understanding what is read) (National Early Literacy Panel, 2008). It is also important to note that oral language plays an important role in learning to read and creative and innovative approaches to learning such as play-based learning strongly support oral language development. During the first years of schooling, the emphasis will be on students learning to read, which should at the very least involve systematic phonics instruction (Hempenstall, 2016). Phonics-based approaches teach children how to match phonemes (sounds) to graphemes (letters). In a synthetic phonics approach, children are systematically introduced to letter sounds (alphabet knowledge), before being taught how to blend these sounds together into syllables and words. It thus utilises a part-to-whole approach: sounding out each letter (e.g. /m/ /o/ /p/) and blending (synthesising) these phonemes into a word (*mop*). Although it goes beyond the scope of this book to provide a detailed overview of this approach, readers are referred to freely accessible publications, such as Hempenstall (2016): *Read about it: Scientific evidence for effective teaching of reading* (see also Parker, 2018) or the Massey University Early Literacy Research Project (https://www.educationcounts.govt.nz/publications/schooling/early-literacy-research-project). It is estimated that, when using an evidence-based approach to early literacy instruction, 90–95% of students will develop accurate and fluent word recognition, with approximately 5–10% of children demonstrating a profile of dyslexia (i.e. specific word reading difficulties), depending on the specific diagnostic criteria that are used (see Al Otaiba, Gillespie Rouse, & Baker, 2018, for a discussion).

1.6.2 The Importance of Early Reading Success

Early success in learning to read is paramount. Apart from the fact that challenges in reading may affect a student's reading self-concept and motivation (e.g. Chapman & Tunmer, 1995), reading ability in first grade is linked to reading ability 10 years later, even after accounting for cognitive ability (Cunningham & Stanovich, 1997). Moreover, failure to develop automatic and fluent word recognition during the early years of schooling will result in less exposure to more complex written texts containing more literate vocabulary (e.g. abstract terms and mental state verbs), more complex grammatical structures, and conforming to more advanced text schemas such as exposition or persuasion. This reduced exposure may in turn hamper the development of more advanced spoken language skills (see case study James in

Chap. 6). This phenomenon where the *'rich get richer and the poor get poorer'* has been coined the Matthew effects in reading (Stanovich, 2009), and highlights the importance of evidence-based reading tuition coupled with early identification and timely remediation of reading difficulties.

1.7   Multi-tiered Systems of Support and Response to Intervention (RtI)

The Response-to-Intervention (RtI) model is a three-tiered framework (Fuchs & Fuchs, 2006) that can be used to guide a school's approach to reading intervention. This model was first introduced in the early 2000s and replaced the more commonly used IQ-achievement discrepancy model in which only students who demonstrated a significant gap between IQ and reading achievement would receive specialist intervention. It basically comprises three tiers.

In Tier 1, all students receive daily high-quality evidence-based reading instruction with effective inclusion of all children through scaffolding and adjustments to support individual student needs. As explained by Denton (2012), instruction should be *differentiated* to ensure the needs of all students in the class are met, as some students may enter school with very low literate cultural capital (i.e. reading-related skills linked to the home literacy environment), whereas others may show high-level reading-related skills (Tunmer, Chapman, & Prochnow, 2006). Moreover, the rate of progression of the curriculum for early reading instruction may simply be too high for some students, particularly those who are at risk of persistent reading difficulties. In the early years of schooling, differentiated instruction should be based on ongoing progress monitoring of student achievement in important foundational skills such as phonological awareness, alphabet knowledge, early word reading skills, and vocabulary.

In Tier 2, those students identified as 'at risk' in Tier 1 (i.e. those who do not make satisfactory progress and are in need of further support) receive supplemental intervention which incorporates pre-teaching and re-teaching of the curriculum, giving students more opportunities to engage in reading instruction, not less. In the early years of reading instruction, Tier 2 intervention will be focused on the constrained skills of phonological awareness, alphabet knowledge and decoding, as well as the unconstrained skills of vocabulary, and/or oral narrative abilities. At the same time as this focused (Tier 2) teaching is being provided, students continue to access the differentiated and explicit teaching planned within the context of the classroom curriculum. It is important that Tier 2 intervention occurs early on in the child's schooling as studies have shown that intervention during the early years of schooling is more effective and time-efficient than intervention during the later years of schooling (see Denton, 2012, for a review). Supplemental intervention is generally provided in small groups, either within or outside the classroom.

In Tier 3, higher intensity reading intervention is provided to those students who do not make satisfactory progress in Tiers 1 and 2. Although the types of activities may be similar to those used in Tier 2, Tier 3 intervention is more intensive and is delivered one-on-one or in small groups. Schools respond to the diverse learning needs of their students by identifying differentiated teaching and learning in all three tiers of planning and instruction.

Fundamental to the RtI model is the use of assessment for cohort mapping, progress monitoring, or reading achievement purposes. Based on the results of these assessments, it can be decided if students make sufficient progress during each level (tier) of intervention. Therefore, ideally, progress monitoring tools need to be easy to administer, time-efficient, sensitive to progress, and appropriate to the local (i.e. Australian) context. In Chap. 2, we will outline the measures we used in this project; in Chap. 3, we will compare them with assessment tools that are commonly used in the schooling system at present.

1.8 Speech-to-Print Profile

To assist educators and other professionals involved in reading to summarise assessment information while ensuring adequate attention is given to the underlying spoken language skills needed for written language, Gillon (2004) introduced the speech-to-print profile. Different professionals involved in the assessment process may use this profile to represent their findings. For example, teachers may collect information related to the student's print concepts, word reading, and phonological awareness skills, whereas speech pathologists may be called upon to conduct more in-depth assessment of a student's spoken language and phonological processing skills. Using the speech-to-print profile will assist collaborative practice, help ensure there is no double-up of assessments, and provide a visual representation of a student's strengths and weaknesses in spoken and written language skills required for successful reading comprehension (see also Gillon, 2018).

The profile contains two main sections: (1) spoken language (underlying representations, phonological awareness, and phonological storage and retrieval) and (2) written language (print knowledge, word level, text level). Because the original profile mainly focused on the underlying spoken language skills needed for word recognition, we adapted the profile (see Table 1.2) to include some important spoken language skills required for reading comprehension (i.e. text-level comprehension including text structure knowledge). We explain the specific assessments that were used to complete these speech-to-print profiles in Chap. 2 and provide case examples in Chap. 6. See Table 1.1 for a brief explanation of some of the terms that are used in the speech-to-print profile, with examples of assessment tasks.

Table 1.2 Speech-to-Print Profile (adapted from Gillon, 2004, with permission from the author)

Spoken language			Written language		
Underlying representations	*Phonological processing*				
Vocabulary knowledge	**Phonological Awareness**	**Storage and Retrieval**	**Rule/concept knowledge**	**Word-level**	**Text-level**
Syntax	*Syllable level*	*Non word repetition*	Print concepts	Word recognition:	*Reading accuracy*
Morphology	*Onset–rime level*	*Multisyllabic word repetition*	Grapheme-Phoneme Correspondences:	*Regular word reading*	*Reading comprehension*
Phonology	*Phoneme level*	*Rapid Naming*	*Single letter*	*Irregular*	*Reading fluency/rate*
Text structure: *Narrative Expository Persuasion*			*Digraph*	*Non-word*	*Writing:*
			Trigraph	Spelling:	
			Diphthongs		

1.9   Evidence-Based Practice from Multiple Perspectives

Reform or change in schools takes time and requires embedded processes in order for sustainable practices to occur. Educational practices and improvements over the past few decades have been swift and enduring (Fullan, 2012), creating extensive pressure on teachers to adapt and adopt new approaches in the classroom. It has been argued that for change within educational contexts, whole-school approaches can be effective in ensuring sustained and positive results (Pendergast et al., 2015). According to Hoare, Bott, and Robinson (2017) "whole-school approaches, being multi-component, collective and collaborative action in the school community, provide optimal opportunity for creating sustained positive change, as opposed to unidimensional, standalone programmes" (p. 59). It is therefore important that whole-school, community approaches are implemented for positive change to result. This means that all parties are involved and invested in making the change work.

Whole-school approaches are driven by strong leadership (Ainscow & Sandill, 2010; Fullan, Hill, & Crévola, 2006; Hill & Crévola, 1997); however, such leadership needs to ensure positive school cultures and quality student outcomes. Barton and McKay (2016) note that "the beliefs of leaders and teachers play a significant role in how they respond to students who experience difficulties with learning" (p. 164) and in particular in relation to reading outcomes. As such, Barton and McKay (2016) offer a model that has at its core the students (see Fig. 1.1).

Significant others in students' lives included in the model include teachers, principals and leadership teams, support staff such as learning support teachers, speech pathologists and other specialists, parents/carers, family, and other community members. All stakeholders are needed to provide the support and encouragement for student success. In the Reading Success project, we recognised the importance of hearing all perspectives (see also Chap. 7).

Fig. 1.1 A whole-school model to support reading (Barton & McKay, 2016). [Permission courtesy of authors]

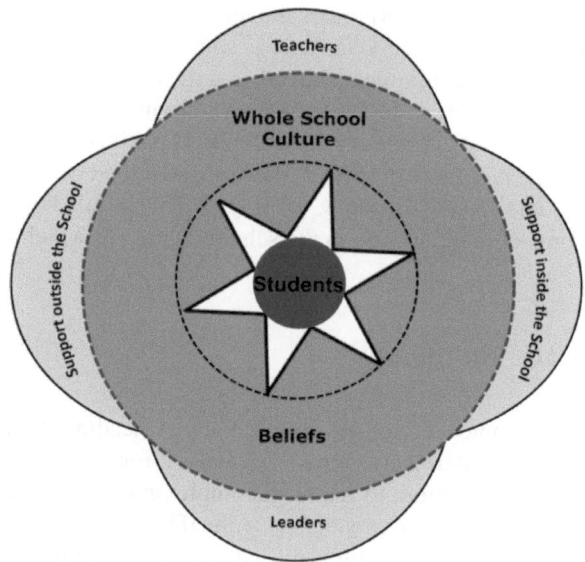

Within this complex space are the big six of reading instruction: phonics, phonological awareness, fluency, comprehension, vocabulary, and oral language (Konza, 2014). Also, as mentioned previously, many other aspects of students' lives impact on learning including students' self-worth, motivation and engagement, cultural and social issues, peers, family and relationships, self-regulation, and affect (see Fig. 1.2).

Fig. 1.2 Understanding the whole learner for effective teaching of reading (Barton & McKay, 2016). [Permission courtesy of authors]

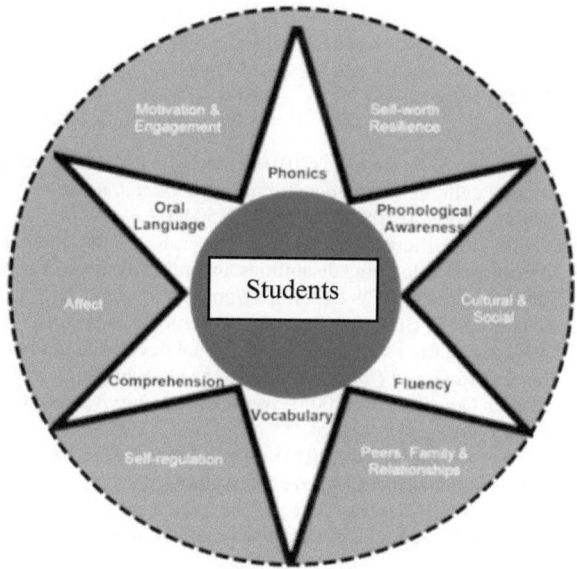

The model incorporates the nature of a whole school's culture, and this includes staff within the school as well as community members. Any approach adopted needs to be well communicated to all, and the benefits that students can gain from people's experience need to be valued. Additionally, the beliefs of teachers, leaders, and support staff in relation to students' capabilities need to be taken into account (see Chap. 4 for more details). If these are stemmed from deficit views, positive outcomes are less likely (Barton & McKay, 2016). In this book, we therefore aim to explore some of these aspects in the school context in which we worked.

1.10 Summary

This chapter defined the Simple View of Reading (SVR) and explained how the SVR can be used as a conceptual framework for categorising both skilled and struggling readers. Learning to read is a complex process and requires both word recognition and language comprehension skills. Difficulties in any of these skills or underlying components may result in difficulties when learning to read. The chapter introduced a range of terms that are frequently used in Australian classrooms including response to intervention (RtI) and multi-tiered systems of support. The use of an evidence-based framework in combination with the adoption of common terminology is important for developing a collaborative approach to the identification and remediation of students at risk for, or experiencing difficulties in reading. Ensuring early reading success and encouraging approaches that support students to enjoy the reading process and share their love for reading with their peers, teachers, and family will result in lifelong positive reading behaviours.

References

Ainscow, M., & Sandill, A. (2010). Developing inclusive education systems: The role of organisational cultures and leadership. *International Journal of Inclusive Education, 14*(4), 401–416. https://doi.org/10.1080/13603110802504903.

Al Otaiba, S., Gillespie Rouse, A., & Baker, K. (2018). Elementary grade intervention approaches to treat specific learning disabilities, including dyslexia. *Language, Speech, and Hearing Services in Schools, 49*(4), 829–842. https://doi.org/10.1044/2018_LSHSS-DYSLC-18-0022.

Amendum, S. J., Bratsch-Hines, M., & Vernon-Feagans, L. (2018). Investigating the efficacy of a web-based early reading and professional development intervention for young English learners. *Reading Research Quarterly, 53*(2), 155–174. https://doi.org/10.1002/rrq.188.

Australian Government. (2005). *Teaching reading: A guide to the report and recommendations for parents and carers.* Author.

Australian Government. (2015). *Action now: Classroom ready teachers. Teacher education ministerial advisory group report.* Author.

Barton, G., & McKay, L. (2016). Conceptualising a literacy education model for junior secondary students: The spatial and reflective practices of an Australian school. *English in Australia, 51*(1), 37–45.

Cain, K., & Oakhill, J. (1996). The nature of the relationship between comprehension skill and the ability to tell a story. *British Journal of Developmental Psychology, 14*, 187–201.

Catts, H. W. (2018). The simple view of reading: Advancements and false impressions. *Remedial and Special Education, 39*(5), 317–323. https://doi.org/10.1177/0741932518767563.

Catts, H. W., Adlof, S. M., & Ellis Weismer, S. (2006). Language deficits in poor comprehenders: A case for the simple view of reading. *Journal of Speech, Language, and Hearing Research, 49*(2), 278–293.

Catts, H. W., Hogan, T. P., & Adlof, S. M. (2005). Developmental changes in reading and reading disabilities. In H. W. Catts & A. G. Kamhi (Eds.), *Connections between language and reading disabilities* (pp. 25–40). Mahwah, NJ: Lawrence Erlbaum.

Catts, H. W., Hogan, T. P., & Fey, M. E. (2003). Subgrouping poor readers on the basis of individual differences in reading-related abilities. *Journal of Learning Disabilities, 36*(2), 151–164. https://doi.org/10.1177/002221940303600208.

Chapman, J. W., & Tunmer, W. E. (1995). Development of young children's reading self-concepts: An examination of emerging subcomponents and their relationship with reading achievement. *Journal of Educational Psychology, 87*(1), 154–167. https://doi.org/10.1037//0022-0663.87.1.154.

Chapman, J. W., & Tunmer, W. E. (2003). Reading difficulties, reading-related self-perceptions, and strategies for overcoming negative self-beliefs. *Reading & Writing Quarterly, 19*(1), 5–24. https://doi.org/10.1080/10573560308205.

Clarke, P. J., Snowling, M. J., Truelove, E., & Hulme, C. (2010). Ameliorating children's reading-comprehension difficulties: A randomized controlled trial. *Psychological Science, 21*(8), 1106–1116.

Cremin, T. (2007). Revisiting reading for pleasure: Delight, desire and diversity. In K. Goouch & A. Lambirth (Eds.), *Understanding phonics and the teaching of reading: A critical perspective* (pp. 166–190). Berkshire, UK: McGraw Hill.

Cremin, T., Mottram, M., Collins, F. M., Powell, S., & Safford, K. (2014). *Building communities of engaged readers: Reading for pleasure*. London: Routledge.

Crystal, D. (1987). Towards a "bucket" theory of language disability: Taking account of interaction between linguistic levels. *Clinical Linguistics and Phonetics, 1*, 7–22.

Cunningham, A. E., & Stanovich, K. E. (1997). Early reading acquisition and its relation to reading experience and ability 10 years later. *Developmental Psychology, 33*(6), 934–945.

Denton, C. A. (2012). Response to Intervention for reading difficulties in the primary grades: Some answers and lingering questions. *Journal of Learning Disabilities, 45*(3), 232–243. https://doi.org/10.1177/0022219412442155.

Fuchs, D., & Fuchs, L. S. (2006). Introduction to response to intervention: What, why, and how valid is it? *Reading Research Quarterly, 41*(1), 93–99. https://doi.org/10.1598/RRQ.41.1.4.

Fullan, M. (2012). *Change forces: Probing the depths of educational reform*. London: Routledge.

Fullan, M., Hill, P., & Crévola, C. (2006). *Breakthrough*. Thousand Oaks, CA: Corwin Press.

Gillon, G. T. (2004). *The speech to print profile*. Christchurch, New Zealand: Author. Profile available from https://www.canterbury.ac.nz/media/documents/education-and-health/gail-gillon—phonological-awareness-resources/resources/speechprintprofile2004.pdf.

Gillon, G. T. (2018). *Phonological awareness: From research to practice* (2nd ed.). New York: The Guilford Press.

Gough, P. B., & Tunmer, W. E. (1986). Decoding, reading, and reading disability. *Remedial and Special Education, 7*(1), 6–10. https://doi.org/10.1177/074193258600700104.

Hempenstall, K. (2016). *Read about it: Scientific evidence for effective teaching of reading CIS research report*. Australia: Centre for Independent Studies.

Hill, P., & Crévola, C. (1997). *Key features of a whole-school, design approach to literacy teaching in schools*. Australia: University of Melbourne.

Hoare, E., Bott, D., & Robinson, J. (2017). Learn it, Live it, Teach it, Embed it: Implementing a whole school approach to foster positive mental health and wellbeing through Positive Education. *International Journal of Wellbeing, 7*(3), 56–71.

Ivey, G. (2014). The social side of engaged reading for young adolescents. *The Reading Teacher,* *68*(3), 165–171.

Justice, L. M. (Ed.). (2006). *Clinical approaches to emergent literacy intervention.* San Diego, CA: Plural Publishing.

Katzir, T., Lesaux, N. K., & Kim, Y.-S. (2009). The role of reading self-concept and home literacy practices in fourth grade reading comprehension. *Reading and Writing, 22*(3), 261–276. https:// doi.org/10.1007/s11145-007-9112-8.

Kintsch, W. (1988). The role of knowledge in discourse comprehension: A construction integration model. *Psychological Review, 95*(2), 163–182.

Konza, D. (2014). Teaching reading: Why the "Fab five" should be the "Big six". *Australian Journal of Teacher Education (Online), 39*(12), 153–169.

Lonigan, C. J., Burgess, S. R., & Schatschneider, C. (2018). Examining the simple view of reading with elementary school children: Still simple after all these years. *Remedial and Special Education, 39*(5), 260–273. https://doi.org/10.1177/0741932518764833.

Marjanovič-Umek, L., Fekonja-Peklaj, U., Sočan, G., & Tašner, V. (2015). A socio-cultural perspective on children's early language: A family study. *European Early Childhood Education Research Journal, 23*(1), 69–85. https://doi.org/10.1080/1350293X.2014.991096.

McGeown, S. P., Duncan, L. G., Griffiths, Y. M., & Stothard, S. E. (2015). Exploring the relationship between adolescents' reading skills, reading motivation and reading habits. *Reading and Writing, 28*(4), 545–569. https://doi.org/10.1007/s11145-014-9537-9.

Mullis, I. V. S., Martin, M. O., Foy, P., & Drucker, K. T. (2012). *PIRLS 2011 International results in reading.* Chestnut Hill, MA, USA: TIMMS & PIRLS International Study Centre.

Nation, K., & Norbury, C. F. (2005). Why reading comprehension fails—Insights from developmental disorders. *Topics in Language Disorders, 25*(1), 21–32.

National Early Literacy Panel. (2008). *Developing early literacy: Report of the National Early Literacy Panel.* Washington, DC: National Institute for Literacy.

NICHD. (2005). Pathways to reading: The role of oral language in the transition to reading. *Developmental Psychology, 41*(2), 428–442.

No Child Left Behind Act. (2002). *20 U.S.C. § 6319.*

Oakhill, J. V., & Cain, K. (2012). The precursors of reading ability in young readers: Evidence from a four-year longitudinal study. *Scientific Studies of Reading, 16*(2), 91–121.

Oakhill, J., Hartt, J., & Samols, D. (2005). Levels of comprehension monitoring and working memory in good and poor comprehenders. *Reading and Writing, 18*(7), 657–686. https://doi.org/ 10.1007/s11145-005-3355-z.

Parker, S. (2018). *Reading instruction and phonics. Theory and practice for teachers.* Boston, MA: Royce-Kotran.

Pendergast, D., Main, K., Barton, G., Kanasa, H., Geelan, D., & Dowden, T. (2015). The Education Change Model as a vehicle for reform: Shifting Year 7 and implementing Junior Secondary in Queensland. *Australian Journal of Middle Schooling.*

Shaywitz, S. E., Shaywitz, B. A., Fletcher, J. M., & Escobar, M. D. (1990). Prevalence of reading disability in boys and girls: Results of the connecticut longitudinal study. *JAMA, 264*(8), 998– 1002. https://doi.org/10.1001/jama.1990.03450080084036.

Snow, C. (2002). *Reading for understanding: Toward an R&D program in reading comprehension.* Santa Monica, CA: Rand Corporation.

Snowling, M. J., & Hulme, C. (2011). Evidence-based interventions for reading and language difficulties: Creating a virtuous circle. *British Journal of Educational Psychology, 81*(1), 1–23. https://doi.org/10.1111/j.2044-8279.2010.02014.x.

Spear-Swerling, L. (2015). *The power of RTI and reading profiles: A blueprint for solving reading problems.* Baltimore, MD: Brookes.

Spear-Swerling, L. (2016). Common types of reading problems and how to help children who have them. *The Reading Teacher, 69*(5), 513–522.

Stanovich, K. E. (2009). Matthew effects in reading: Some consequences of individual differences in the acquisition of literacy. *Journal of Education, 189*(1–2), 23–55.

Stark, H. L., Snow, P. C., Eadie, P. A., & Goldfeld, S. R. (2016). Language and reading instruction in early years' classrooms: the knowledge and self-rated ability of Australian teachers. *Annals of Dyslexia, 66*(1), 28–54. https://doi.org/10.1007/s11881-015-0112-0.

Stein, N., & Glenn, C. (1979). An analysis of story comprehension in elementary school children. In R. O. Freedle (Ed.), *New directions in discourse processing* (Vol. 2, pp. 53–120). Norwood, NJ: Ablex.

Thompson, R., & Whimper, L. A. (2010). Exposure to family violence and reading level of early adolescents. *Journal of Aggression, Maltreatment & Trauma, 19*(7), 721–733. https://doi.org/10.1080/10926771003781347.

Tunmer, W. E., Chapman, J. W., & Prochnow, J. E. (2006). Literate cultural capital at school entry predicts later reading achievement: A seven year longitudinal study. *New Zealand Journal of Educational Studies, 41*(2), 183–204.

Tunmer, W. E., & Hoover, W. A. (2019). The cognitive foundations of learning to read: A framework for preventing and remediating reading difficulties. *Australian Journal of Learning Difficulties, 24*(1), 75–93. https://doi.org/10.1080/19404158.2019.1614081.

Verhoeven, L., & van Leeuwe, J. (2012). The simple view of second language reading throughout the primary grades. *Reading and Writing, 25*(8), 1805–1818. https://doi.org/10.1007/s11145-011-9346-3.

Westerveld, M. F., Gillon, G. T., & Moran, C. (2008). A longitudinal investigation of oral narrative skills in children with mixed reading disability. *International Journal of Speech-Language Pathology, 10*(3), 132–145. https://doi.org/10.1080/14417040701422390.

Woolley, G. (2011). *Reading comprehension: Assisting children with learning difficulties.* Dordrecht, NLD: Springer.

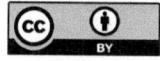

Part I
The Reading Success Project

Chapter 2
Methodology

Marleen F. Westerveld, Rebecca M. Armstrong, and Georgina M. Barton

Abstract This chapter describes the methodology used in the Reading Success project. We start by briefly describing the school's context, including the student cohorts who were involved in the project. The specific qualitative data collection methods relating to existing school initiatives for improving the reading performance of their students are then described. The second half of this chapter outlines the assessment process, including a brief explanation of the types of assessments that can be used (formal vs. informal; standardised vs. criterion-referenced) and how to interpret these types of assessment results. We then describe the five-step assessment process we used to determine which students showed challenges in aspects of their spoken and/or written language skills to determine which students might benefit from specific intervention to address their reading needs. An overview of the specific assessment tasks that were used to determine the students' performance at each step of the process is included along with a clear rationale for each assessment and an explanation of how these assessment results map on to the speech-to-print profile. Finally, consideration is given to progress monitoring practices.

Keywords Reading assessment · Speech-to-print profile · Progress monitoring

2.1 A Brief Overview of the School Involved in the Reading Success Project

The Australian school involved in the Reading Success project identified the assessment and intervention practices for reading as a major area for school improvement. At the time of completing the project, there were 674 students (50% males/50% females) enrolled at the school. These enrolments included 6% of students who identified as being indigenous and 31% of students who had a language background other than English. The Index of Community Socio-Educational Advantage (ICSEA) scale (Australian Curriculum, Assessment and Reporting Authority [ACARA], n.d.) was used as an indicator of the demographic composition of the school. ICSEA is a scale developed by ACARA and used to provide an indication of the level of educational advantage of students attending the school. An overall ICSEA value is calculated for each school, based on factors including parents' occupation, parents'

© The Author(s) 2020

M. F. Westerveld et al., *Reading Success in the Primary Years*,

https://doi.org/10.1007/978-981-15-3492-8_2

education, a school's geographical location, and the proportion of indigenous students. The average ICSEA score (or the benchmark) is 1000, with scores falling between approximately 500 (representing students from extremely disadvantaged backgrounds) and 1300 (representing students from more advantaged backgrounds). The school involved in this project had a school ICSEA value of 1005 suggesting the level of educational advantage for this school was consistent with the average benchmark across Australia. However, it should be noted that according to the Australian Early Development Census data (https://www.aedc.gov.au/ 2015 data), the proportion of children attending the school who were considered developmentally vulnerable in language and cognitive skills was double in comparison with the reported percentage of children considered developmentally vulnerable residing in the school's geographic region.

In Australia, the National Assessment Program—Literacy and Numeracy (NAPLAN) is a nationwide assessment process undertaken in all Australian schools with students in Years 3, 5, 7, and 9 (Australian Government, 2016). The assessment is designed to test the types of skills that are essential for every child to progress through school and life, including skills in reading, writing, spelling, grammar and punctuation, and numeracy. Students are provided with individual results explaining their performance on NAPLAN; however, schools also gain information relating to their overall school performance. Through using ICSEA, schools are able to compare their performance to that of other schools with similar educational advantage values. For the school in the current project, it was evident that their reading results on NAPLAN showed that on average the students performed similar to students attending similar schools over time, despite the school facing many unique challenges.

The Reading Success project included all key stakeholders involved in the teaching of reading in the school setting, resulting in an interdisciplinary approach to both the identification of reading difficulties and the provision of targeted intervention for students at risk of or experiencing difficulties in reading. As part of this collaborative approach, qualitative data and reports obtained from the school leadership team, teachers, and students were included. Reading achievement data collected from two cohorts of students at different stages of their reading development will be reported on in this book:

The Learning to Read stage Students in the 'learning to read' phase of development included students in Year 1 (i.e. their second year of formal schooling). Parents of 94% (93 out of 99 students) of the overall Year 1 cohort provided consent for their child to be involved in this project, providing a representative sample of all students in Year 1 at this school. Of these students, 46% were male, and 32% spoke a language other than English in the home environment (E/ALD) as determined based on parent report data.

The Reading to Learn stage Students in the 'reading to learn' phase of development included students in Year 4 (i.e. their fifth year of formal schooling). A total of 83% (78 out of 94 students) of the overall Year 4 cohort was involved in this project, providing a representative sample of all students in Year 4 at this school. Of these students, 47% were male, and 24% had E/ALD as determined based on parent report data.

The specific data collection methods for both the qualitative aspect of this project and the data pertaining to reading achievement are described in further detail below.

2.2   Stakeholder Interviews

To obtain information about the educators' perspectives about their school as well as their opinions about the enablers and/or inhibitors of the school's reading programmes and approaches to the teaching of reading, a number of qualitative data sets were collected to ensure richness of the data (Lambert & Loiselle, 2008):

> a productive iterative process whereby an initial model of the phenomenon guided the exploration of individual accounts and successive individual data further enriched the conceptualisation of the phenomenon; identification of the individual and contextual circumstances surrounding the phenomenon, which added to the interpretation of the structure of the phenomenon; and convergence of the central characteristics of the phenomenon across focus groups and individual interviews, which enhanced trustworthiness of findings. (p. 228)

Therefore, the qualitative data included in the Reading Success project were collected through interviews and/or focus groups with teachers (at the beginning and at the end of the project), interviews with the leadership team, and a student focus group as well as individual student interviews. Information was also collected about the reading programmes the school implemented over the course of the project. In addition, school planning documents and policies were included in the data set.

Educators The interview questions for teachers and leaders firstly focused on their demographics—how long they had been teaching, what their qualifications were, and what year levels they had taught previously including any other teaching experiences. Remaining questions explored what the educators' perspectives were about their school as well as what they felt were the enablers and/or inhibitors of the school's reading programmes and approaches to the teaching of reading. The post-interviews also investigated what staff members felt about the Reading Success project including its impact on student learning. Prompt questions for both the pre- and post-interviews can be found in Appendix 1. The questions were based on a previous project conducted by Barton and McKay (2014, 2016a, 2016b) that explored another school's approach to teaching reading in the secondary context.

Students The student focus group and subsequent interviews involved students in the *reading to learn* cohort (i.e. Year 4 students). Three of these students rated themselves the lowest on the *Reading Self-Concept Scale* (Chapman & Tunmer, 1995). Initially, the students were invited as a whole group to participate in a focus group to talk about reading, how they perceive themselves as readers and what might help or inhibit their reading. While the students participated in this focus group, the researcher asked them to create a collage using cut-up pictures from a range of magazines. The purpose of this collage was to support the students in feeling comfortable about talking about themselves with the researcher. The researcher utilised a method known as *re-collage* (Barton, 2020), whereby participants create an artwork that expresses deeper messages about a topic, in this case reading. Arts-based research methods have been known to support participants' abilities to express their feelings about focused topics. For students of this age, the researchers were interested in not only asking for their opinions orally, but also using a stimulus artwork created by the participants to base a discussion around.

Allowing the students to reflect on themselves as readers through the art had potential for students to uncover aspects of themselves as readers not previously known. Leitch (2006), for example, explained that "*through the creation of images in relation to self, new meanings, previously unaware, unvoiced, unexpressed, half-understood came to be significant and capable of being incorporated into the participants' social and/or emotional understanding of themselves, to the point that new actions or directions could be taken in their lives*" (p. 566). In a similar vein, McNiff (2008) showed how arts-based and creative approaches to reflecting on a topic often resulted in more "meaningful insights [that] often come by surprise, unexpectedly and even against the will of the creator" (p. 40). Utilising modes, other than language, created the opportunity for the students to feel safe and express different ways of knowing or being (Liamputtong & Rumbold, 2008).

Analytical approaches All interviews and focus groups were audio recorded and then transcribed. Participants were provided with the transcripts in order for member checking to occur. The team then analysed the transcripts by firstly identifying any codes (interesting factors) throughout the initial reading of documents. Subsequently, the team re-read each transcript to ensure no code was left unidentified. Finally, the codes were clustered into identified themes (Braun & Clarke, 2006). The identified themes from the educator and student perspectives are described in detail in Chaps. 4 and 7.

2.3   Student Reading Self-Concept

As outlined in Chap. 1, student self-perception/motivation for reading is an important aspect to consider when creating reading profiles and when planning for intervention (Cartwright, Marshall, & Wray, 2016; Katzir, Lesaux, & Kim, 2009). For this reason, students in the *reading to learn* cohort completed the *Reading Self-Concept Scale* (Chapman & Tunmer, 1995) as part of this project. This scale comprises 30 items to determine students' self-perceptions across three different subscales: (1) perception of their competency in reading, (2) perception of reading difficulty, and (3) their attitudes towards reading. For each item, the statement is read aloud to the child by the examiner. This oral administration ensures reading skills of the child do not impact on completion of the task. If the student does not understand any of the questions, the examiner provides further explanation related to the statement. The student is then required to respond to each statement on a five-point scale ranging from '*Yes, always*' to '*No, never*'. Student responses are scored from 1 (indicating a low reading self-concept) to 5 (indicating a high reading self-concept) and then summed to provide an overall score based on the 30 responses. Comparisons between the child's responses across the three different subscales can also be conducted. Student performance on this scale is described in Chap. 4.

2.4 Types of Assessments and Interpretation of Results

2.4.1 Assessment Type

In selecting assessments to complete the speech-to-print profile and describe a student's strengths and weaknesses in the skills needed for successful reading, it is important to understand the underlying features and components of different tests and how these features may influence the information that can be obtained. Broadly speaking, assessments can be formal or informal in design (see Table 2.1). Formal assessments are standardised, which means that they are well constructed, and have clear administration and scoring processes to ensure that administration of the assessment is 'standard' no matter who administers the test or scores it. Most formal assessments are norm-referenced, which means that a student's performance can be compared to his/her same-age or same-grade peers. Informal assessments, on the other hand, are often less structured and contextualised (more authentic) and can include observational assessments, screening assessments, interviews, and questionnaires. Informal assessment tasks are not standardised, and do not have norms. This means that although a student's performance can be observed and described, it is not possible to compare the student's performance to his/her peers. Both formal and informal assessments may be criterion-referenced. This type of assessment is different from norm-referenced tests, as the focus is on determining whether the child can achieve a certain level of performance (rather than comparing a child with the performance of another). This type of assessment has advantages as it examines behaviours in depth and can be a useful method for establishing baseline performance and monitoring treatment progress.

2.4.2 Interpretation of Norm-Referenced Test Results

The features of standardisation for norm-referenced assessments allow for student performance to be compared with other students (i.e. the norming sample) who are the same age or the same year of schooling, and their strengths and difficulties can be interpreted accordingly. More specifically, student performance on standardised assessments can be interpreted using a bell curve (see Fig. 2.1). A bell curve is a representation of normal distribution and shows that the further a person's score moves away from the mean (in either direction) the fewer people in the population will receive that score. Most standardised tests report mean scores for each age group and also a standard deviation. The standard deviation represents the average

Table 2.1 An overview of different types of assessments

Formal = standardised	Informal = non-standardised	
Prescribed and well-defined procedures for administering and scoring of the test Psychometric properties of assessment are reported	Provides a less structured, more natural approach to measuring or observing performance	
Norm-referenced	Criterion-referenced	Authentic
• Diagnostic • Always standardised • Comparison with same-age/same-grade students • Allows for comparisons across different standardised assessments testing different skills (e.g. oral language and reading) • Decontextualised	• Identify what a student can/cannot do compared to predetermined criterion • Does not compare to other students • Some opportunity for individualisation • May be diagnostic	• Identify what a student can/cannot do • Emphasis is on contextualised stimuli (i.e. conducted in realistic environment) • May be ongoing; completed across both assessment and treatment contexts
Reporting examples (phonological awareness assessment task)		
The student's performance on a standardised phonological awareness test = standard score 85. This means the student scores 1 standard deviation below his peers (same year of schooling)	The student is able to identify initial sounds in words—this is expected at the student's level of schooling (i.e. middle of year 1)	During a shared book reading activity, the student was able to provide three other words that rhymed with /man/, but could not provide any other words that started with a /m/ sound

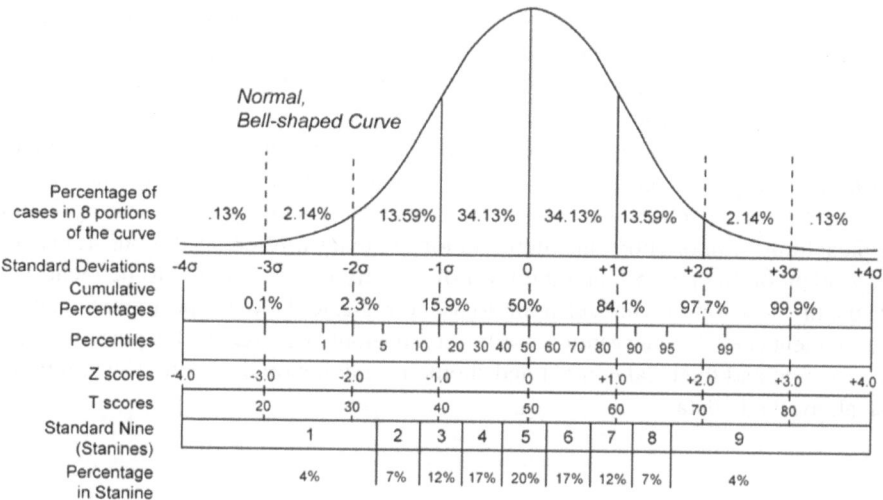

Fig. 2.1 Bell curve. (*Source* Wikimedia Commons, retrieved from https://commons.wikimedia. org/wiki/Category:Normal_distribution#/media/File:Normal_distribution_and_scales.gif)

difference of scores from the mean score to account for variability that exists in test scores amongst different test takers. It is the combination of information from the mean and standard deviation of a test that allows decisions to be made about when a child's score falls far enough from the mean to warrant the decision that it is significantly different from the norm. Raw scores (i.e. the total number of items the student got correct on a standardised test) need to be converted to allow for meaningful comparisons to norms provided for each test. These comparisons result in the creation of standard scores (such as z-scores or scaled scores) or percentile ranks which can be used to provide an indication of how far from the mean the child performs on a test in comparison with the normative data for that assessment. The interpretation of these three types of scores, z-scores, scaled scores, and percentile ranks is provided below.

Z-scores A z-score of 0 indicates average performance (see Fig. 2.1), with a negative score indicating performance below the mean and a positive score falling above the mean. A student's performance with a z-score below -1 indicates the child's performance is more than 1 standard deviation below the mean and is subsequently interpreted as performing 'below expectations'.

Scaled Scores The interpretation of scaled scores, or standard scores, is usually based on the mean score that is assigned for each test. For example, it is common for tests to assign a mean score of 100 (i.e. z-score of 0), and scores less than 85 indicate a child's performance is more than 1 standard deviation below the mean, and thus 'below expectations'.

Percentile Rank A percentile rank refers to the proportion of the normative population that scored lower than the subject taking the test. A percentile rank of less than 16 is indicative of performance 1 standard deviation below the mean, suggesting skills 'below expectations'.

The bell curve in Fig. 2.1 provides a visual representation of the association of all these types of scores. In Fig. 2.1, you can see that 68.2% of the population scores between z-scores -1 and $+1$ and hence is considered to be scoring within typical limits. Importantly, the interpretation of all norm-referenced scores is usually dependent on the purpose and the level of severity that is required to be identified. Thus, the decision of what cut-point to use to indicate 'below expectations' and the subsequent need for intervention is arbitrary. It should be based on the purpose of the assessment and the local context and should be a collaborative team decision based on all available data.

2.5   Choosing a Reading Comprehension Test

As stated previously, the aim of learning to read is to read *accurately* and *fluently* with *comprehension*. To determine the level of reading ability, it is therefore important to use a formal reading assessment that adequately captures a student's reading skills across reading accuracy, reading fluency, and reading comprehension. As summarised by Westerveld (2009), when choosing a reading comprehension test, the following needs to be taken into consideration: (1) test format (i.e. cloze vs question–answer format; oral or silent); (2) passage dependency (can the students answer the questions without reading the passage); and (3) test-taking strategies (i.e. student initiative, involvement, and item completion rate; Bornholt, 2002; Keenan & Betjemann, 2006; Keenan, Betjemann, & Olson, 2008).

Unfortunately, not all reading tests adequately measure reading *comprehension*. In fact, some assessments may fail to identify reading comprehension deficits (Bowyer-Crane & Snowling, 2005). For example, student performance based on tests such as the *Neale Analysis of Reading Ability* (NARA; Neale, 1999) and the *York Assessment of Reading for Comprehension* (YARC; Snowling et al., 2012) depends on both word recognition and language comprehension skill, as students are asked to answer questions after readig a passage. In contrast, performance on cloze reading tasks (i.e. student reads a sentence or passage and fills in the blank) has been shown to be mostly dependent on adequate word recognition ability. Based on these results, Westerveld (2009) advised the use of a reading test that requires the student to read passages and answer open-ended questions following the reading or using an individually administered test of language comprehension in addition to using a reading test (Nation & Snowling, 1997).

Another consideration in the Australian context is to choose a test that has been normed on the Australian population. Recognising the importance of the schooling system, including the effect of what age students start their formal reading tuition (Cunningham & Carroll, 2011) on their reading performance, using standardised tests that have been normed overseas may not adequately identify Australian students with reading difficulties. Both the NARA and the YARC have been normed on Australian students. A recent study by Colenbrander, Nickels, and Kohnen (2016) compared student performance on the NARA versus the YARC. Students attended Australian primary schools and were in grades 3–6. Interestingly, more students were classified with a 'specific comprehension difficulty' profile on the NARA than on the YARC, but no differences were found for classification of 'specific word reading difficulties' between the tests. Closer inspection of these results, however, showed that only 9% of the variance in YARC scores could be explained by a child's ability to decode words; this was 21% for the NARA. Taken together, the authors concluded that the YARC may be a better test to indicate reading comprehension difficulties for students who have word recognition difficulties. Furthermore, the authors recommend using a separate decoding task (word or non-word reading measure), and that diagnosis of a reading comprehension difficulty should not be based on the results of a single assessment. For the current study, based on previous research, we administered the YARC to determine students' reading performance across reading accuracy, reading fluency, and reading comprehension.

2.6 The Reading Assessment Process Used in the Reading Success Project

As part of the Reading Success project, comprehensive assessments of students' reading and spoken language skills were undertaken to create speech-to-print profiles for those students who struggled with their reading comprehension. As explained in Chap. 1, this assessment process was guided by the Simple View of Reading (SVR) as a framework and included several steps to determine individual reading profiles, which in turn were used to inform intervention practices. First, students' reading comprehension performance was assessed using a standardised, norm-referenced reading assessment (Step 1). Next, for students with identified reading comprehension difficulties, their skills in reading accuracy and language comprehension were assessed (Step 2). For those students with identified difficulties in reading accuracy, additional testing to determine proficiency in word recognition skills (including single word reading, orthographic knowledge, and phonological awareness) was conducted (Step 3). Finally, for each student who scored below expectations on reading comprehension in Step 1, individual speech-to-print profiles were created to visually represent the assessment data and show: (1) strengths and weaknesses in the underlying spoken language skills needed for successful reading performance and (2) strengths and weaknesses in the code-related skills needed for successful word

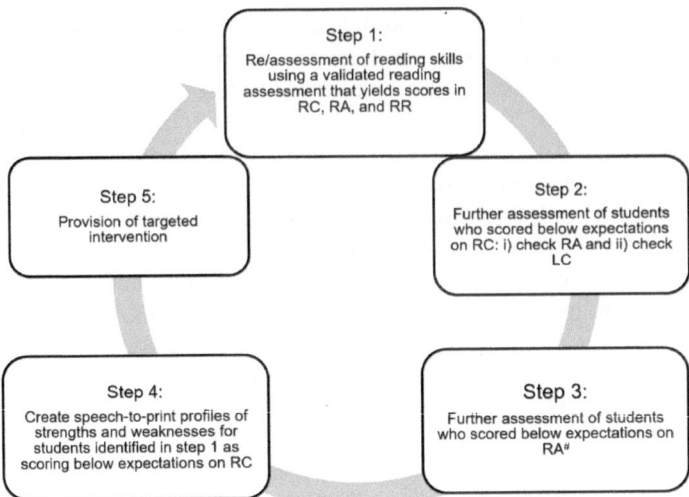

Fig. 2.2 Five-step assessment to intervention process based on the Simple View of Reading. *Note* RC = Reading comprehension; RA = reading accuracy; RR = reading rate; LC = language comprehension. [#]Step 3: Further assessment may also include students whose RC was within expectations but their RA was below expectations and may warrant further assessment (see Step 3 below)

recognition (Step 4). Finally, the information obtained from Steps 1–4 was used to guide intervention practices as part of Step 5. This assessment to intervention process is shown descriptively in Fig. 2.2.

The following section details these five assessment steps including description of the specific assessments administered as part of the Reading Success project. We acknowledge that there are many other assessments available to assess reading and spoken language skills of school-aged children and recommend collaboration with all professionals involved in assessment and intervention for students at risk for or experiencing difficulties in reading, including speech pathologists. The tests that were used in this project are described in detail below; however, a list of other suitable tests are shown as further examples in Appendix 2.

2.6.1   Step 1: Assessment of Reading Skills Using a Validated Assessment

For this project, the Australian edition of the *York Assessment of Reading for Comprehension, Primary* (YARC; Snowling et al., 2012), was used as a formal (standardised), norm-referenced assessment of reading ability. The YARC yields measures of reading accuracy and reading comprehension as well as reading rate. This diagnostic reading assessment was administered individually, either by a speech pathologist or by a teacher, with all students in the project. As per the manual, the student was asked to read aloud two passages (at a level suitable to the student's reading ability), and the time taken to read each passage was recorded. If the student produced a reading error, the correct production was immediately provided to the student by the examiner. At the conclusion of each passage, the student was asked a series of literal and inferential comprehension questions, and the student was able to refer to the text to answer the questions if they needed. Following the completion of two passages, several scores were calculated: (a) the number of reading errors was totalled to provide an overall reading accuracy (RA) score; (b) the time taken to read each passage was summed to provide an overall reading rate (RR); (c) the total number of questions answered correctly was calculated to provide a reading comprehension (RC) score. These raw scores were then converted to standard scores to allow for comparisons with Australian normative data. As per the test guidelines, for students in the Year 1 cohort, RR was not calculated if the student exceeded 16 reading errors on the level 1 passage. These test scores (RA, RR, and RC) can be calculated online using a free online score conversion tool.

In the Reading Success project, we used a standard score (SS) cut-off of 85 as an indicator of 'below expectations', which corresponds to students scoring in the bottom 16% of the same-age population (see Fig. 2.1). Using this cut-off, the cohort was divided into those students who needed further assessment and those who performed within expectations for their age/stage of schooling.

2.6.2 Step 2: Further Assessment of Students Who Scored Below Expectations on Reading Comprehension

For students who scored below expectations on the RC subtest of the YARC, consistent with the Simple View of Reading, we investigated their reading accuracy skills and considered their language comprehension skills.

(i) **Check Reading Accuracy** First, student performance on the YARC RA subtest was checked to determine whether challenges in RA were contributing to RC difficulties. Students who demonstrated RA SS < 85 were considered to demonstrate challenges in RA.

(ii) **Check Language Comprehension** The next step was to screen the language comprehension skills of students who scored below expectations in RC. In this project the *Understanding Spoken Paragraphs* subtest from the standardised, norm-referenced assessment, the *Clinical Evaluation of Language Fundamentals*, fourth or fifth edition (CELF-4/CELF-5; Semel, Wiig, & Secord, 2006; Wiig, Semel, & Secord, 2017) was administered. As per the test manual, students were asked to listen to spoken passages and then answer questions about the content of the passages. The subtest was administered as per the assessment manual guidelines, and a total raw score was calculated and then converted to a scaled score. In the current project, a scaled score below 7, i.e. 1

standard deviation below the mean, was used to indicate a student performing 'below expectations' in language comprehension (i.e. equivalent to SS85).

The CELF is a restricted test (i.e. can only be administered by a speech pathologist) and is relatively expensive if the only aim of using it is to determine if the student's RC difficulties stem from underlying problems in LC. An alternative way of assessing LC is to orally administer two paragraphs of the YARC. The YARC Passage Reading Test—Primary comprises two parallel tests of graded passages (A and B), each of which is accompanied by a set of eight comprehension questions. Therefore, if form A has been used to test the student's RC, form B can be used to test the student's LC. In this instance, the examiner (e.g. teacher or speech pathologist) reads two passages (level equivalent to the student's age or year of schooling) out loud and asks the student to answer the comprehension questions afterwards. The student's performance can be evaluated by scoring the total number of questions answered correctly across the two passages and converting this raw score to a scaled score. Although this test was not normed for this purpose, a scaled score $\geq$ 85 would potentially indicate satisfactory language comprehension performance.

The results from Steps 1 and 2 were then used to determine whether students' poor performance on the RC subtest of the YARC could be explained by poor RA, poor LC, or both.

2.6.3 Step 3: Further Assessment of Word Recognition Skills

Next, for students who performed below expectations in RA on the YARC (i.e. showed difficulties accurately reading passages), further assessment was conducted to determine possible underlying reasons for their RA difficulties. It is important to note that assessment at this stage should include students who demonstrate poor RA and RC (both SS < 85), as well as those students whose RC SS $\geq$ 85 but who show difficulties in RA (i.e. SS < 85). This is an important consideration as these students, who demonstrate decoding difficulties but age-appropriate RC, may have oral language skills that allow for masking of difficulties in RC, particularly in the early years of schooling. Therefore, further assessment of these students' word recognition skills and consideration of targeted intervention around decoding may be required.

Assessments of the following print-related skills were conducted: (a) single word reading, (b) orthographic knowledge, and (c) phonological awareness.

Single Word Reading

The *Castles and Coltheart Word Reading Test*—Second Edition (CC-2; Castles, et al., 2009) was administered as a formal, standardised, norm-referenced measure of single word reading ability. This test was selected as it has Australian normative data, is freely available, and is an efficient measure of word reading across regular, irregular, and nonsense words. This test is untimed and assesses a student's ability to read aloud a series of single words, including 40 regular, 40 irregular, and 40 nonsense words. This test was administered online according to the test guidelines, and the words were presented one at a time, in a pseudo-randomised order, and with gradually increasing difficulty. Once a student makes > 5 errors on any of the single word subtypes, the administration of that subtype is discontinued. The student continues with the remaining word types until the ceiling is reached for all subtypes or until all words have been read. A total raw accuracy score for each subtest type (regular, irregular, and nonsense words) was calculated and then converted to a z-score for the child's age. A z-score below -1 indicated a student performing below expectations on single word reading ability.

Orthographic Knowledge

The *Letter Sound Test* (LeST; Larsen, Kohnen, Nickels, & McArthur, 2015) assessed orthographic knowledge. This freely available, formal, norm-referenced assessment was chosen to assess a student's ability to sound out single letters and letter combinations (including consonant and vowel digraphs). The test has been normed on Australian students (kindergarten to grade 3). This test was administered online (www.motif.org.au), in a one-to-one setting, and took approximately 5–10 min. Students were shown 51 graphemes (single letters and letter combinations) in isolation, and they were asked to produce the target sound . After the administration of the test, a total raw score (/51) was calculated and converted to a z-score as per the test guidelines. In the current study, students with a z-score less than -1 were classified as performing below expectations with their orthographic knowledge, including the students attending Year 4 who were older than the norming sample.

Phonological Awareness

The *Sutherland Phonological Awareness Test—Revised* (SPAT-R; Neilson, 2003) was administered to assess the students' phonological awareness skills. This standardised test was normed on 559 Australian students, is suitable for students in their first to fourth year of schooling, and takes approximately 10–15 min to administer. For students in Year 1, the first seven subtests of the SPAT-R were administered individually according to the test manual instructions. The first seven subtests provided an indication of phonological awareness skills in terms of syllable segmentation, rhyme detection and production, blending and segmenting phonemes, and onset–rime identification. All subtests involved the students completing four items for each task. In this project, subtest scores below the 25th percentile were used to identify students whose phonological awareness skills were below expectations and potentially of concern.

For older students, in Step 3 of the assessment process, we used subtests from the *Comprehensive Test of Phonological Processing—Second Edition* (CTOPP-2; Wagner, Torgesen, & Rashotte, 2013), including: (a) elision, measuring a student's ability to remove segments from spoken words to form other words; i.e. phoneme awareness; (b) non-word repetition; (c) rapid automatic naming; and (d) non-word repetition. The CTOPP-2 is a restricted test (i.e. only allied health and special education professionals can administer this test).

2.6.4 Step 4: Creating Speech-to-Print Profiles

Table 2.2 provides an overview of the assessments that were used in Steps 1–3. Speech-to-print profiles were created for students who performed below expectation on the RC subtest of the YARC. Information from all assessment measures (from Steps 1 to 3) was mapped on to the speech-to-print profiles for each student. It is paramount to ensure this step of the assessment process is in collaboration with all stakeholders involved in the teaching and remediation of reading, including teachers, speech pathologists, and learning support teachers. This collaborative process allows for the identification of strengths and difficulties in the core components of language comprehension and word recognition. Furthermore, this team approach provides an avenue for identifying if any further assessments should be completed and by whom, or whether some of this information has already been collected as part of routine school-wide assessment processes. For example, as shown in Table 2.2, Step 4 may require a comprehensive evaluation of a student's spoken language skills, which may involve a referral to the speech pathologist. The speech pathologist may, for example, administer the CELF-5 and/or collect a spontaneous language sample in a narrative (e.g. Profile of Oral Narrative Ability [PONA]; Westerveld & Vidler, 2016) or expository context (Heilmann & Malone, 2014). For other students, more detailed information may be needed regarding a student's writing and spelling skills, which may well be available from the classroom teacher. Completing the profile will then promote discussion about appropriate intervention planning (see Step 5).

2.6.5 Step 5: Provision of Targeted Intervention

The next step was to discuss how appropriate and targeted intervention could be provided for students with identified reading difficulties, based on their speech-to-print profiles. For example students who showed a profile of dyslexia would benefit from intervention aimed at improving these students' phonological processing and word recognition skills, whereas students who demonstrated specific comprehension deficits would benefit from a programme aimed at improving their language comprehension skills. In this project, the speech-to-print profiles were discussed with the school team to: (1) trial appropriate interventions for a selection of students within the school setting, and (2) allow for the school team to plan and continue to implement regular classroom instruction. Detailed information about the interventions implemented and evaluated as part of the Reading Success project is provided in Chap. 5. Case samples are presented in Chap. 6.

Table 2.2   An overview of the areas assessed and the assessment methods used at each step

	Area to assess	Assessment used	Skill	Type of assessment
Step 1	Reading comprehension (text level)	YARC—form A	Student's ability to answer questions from a passage of text that they had read	Standardised, norm-referenced (scaled scores)
Step 2 i	Reading accuracy (text level)	YARC—form A	Student's ability to accurately read aloud a passage of text	Standardised, norm-referenced (scaled scores)
Step 2 ii	Language comprehension (text level)	CELF-4/CELF-5 *Understanding Spoken Paragraphs* Or use the YARC—form B	Student's ability to answer comprehension questions after listening to short passages	Standardised, norm-referenced (scaled scores)
Step 3	Word recognition (word level)	CC-2 (Motif)	Student's ability to read aloud single words of different word types including: regular, irregular, and nonsense words	Standardised, norm-referenced (z-score)
	Grapheme–phoneme correspondences	LeST (Motif)	Student's ability to produce sound to a corresponding letter /letter combination	Standardised, norm-referenced (z-score)
	Phonological awareness	SPAT-R	Student's ability to complete syllable, rhyme, and phoneme identification tasks	Standardised, norm-referenced (percentile ranks)
		CTOPP-2	Phonological processing, including phoneme awareness, rapid automatic naming, and non-word repetition	Standardised, norm-referenced (standard scores)

(continued)

Table 2.2 (continued)

	Area to assess	Assessment used	Skill	Type of assessment
Step 4	Spoken language: Vocabulary Syntax Morphology	CELF-4/CELF-5 Core Language Subtests	Student's ability to complete core subtests tapping semantic, syntactic, morphological knowledge	Standardised, norm-referenced. Standard score
	Text structure knowledge	Profile of Oral Narrative Ability (PONA)	Student's ability to retell a well-sequenced coherent narrative	Formal (using a protocol). Norms for students in Prep and Year 1
		Expository Scoring Scheme	Student's ability to produce a well-sequenced, coherent, and informative explanation of a game or sport	Formal (using a protocol), but not normed for this age range

2.7   Progress Monitoring

As explained in Chap. 1, progress monitoring underpins the response-to-intervention framework. Monitoring of student progress was conducted on a regular basis as part of normal school procedures, and more in-depth assessment of reading and spoken language skills was undertaken following periods of targeted (Tier 2 and Tier 3) intervention. Examples of progress monitoring practices are described next.

2.7.1   School-initiated Assessments for Reading

The school utilised several routine data collection methods for monitoring reading outcomes across the school years. The following section describes these specific methods; however, it is important to note that other Australian schools would have different processes for measuring reading outcomes. At the school where the Reading Success project was undertaken, it was reported by the school leadership team that the assessments administered change throughout primary school based on student year level and reading level. In the early foundational years of schooling, the *PM Benchmark Reading Assessment Resource Kit* (Smith, Nelley, & Croft, 2009) was used to measure reading skills. Once the students exceeded the maximum reading level on the PM Benchmark (i.e. level 30), teachers administered the *Prose Reading*

Observation Behaviour & Evaluation of Comprehension—Second Edition (PROBE 2; Parkin & Parkin, 2011) and the *Progressive Achievement Tests in Reading* (PAT-R; Australian Council for Educational Research, 2018). Further information about these assessment tools is provided next.

Learning to Read Cohort The PM Benchmark assesses students' instructional and independent reading levels using levelled fiction and non-fiction texts. The assessment is criterion-referenced, is administered individually, and takes approximately 15–20 min to complete per student. There are different reading levels which are expected for each year level to determine 'average' and 'below average' reading performance. The highest level obtainable is level 30. The final reading level is based on the student's performance in decoding, retelling, and answering comprehension questions. At early levels, these comprehension questions are literal, and as students progress through the reading levels both literal and inferential questions are included. At the school where this project was conducted, students in the early years of schooling were assessed on the PM Benchmark every term as part of the school's process for tracking reading progress.

Reading to Learn Cohort The PROBE 2 and PAT-R are two reading comprehension assessments that are commonly used in Queensland schools. As the PROBE is organised across six-month developmental intervals, it is not sensitive enough to measure progress each term. Therefore, once students reached a PM Benchmark level of 30, the school alternated between administration of the PROBE 2 and the PAT-R.

The PAT-R is a norm-referenced test of reading comprehension and can be used with students in Prep to Year 10. It takes approximately 40 min to administer plus 15 min for scoring. However, the test can be administered and scored online, automatically generating a range of reports, including group reports and individual reports. The test yields scaled scores, percentile rank scores, and stanines.

The PROBE 2 consists of 20 sets (one fiction and one non-fiction passage) of graded passages with reading ages ranging from 5 to 6 years to 14.5–15.5 years. The test should be administered individually and takes about 15–20 min. The examiner estimates the starting level and asks the student to first read the passage silently and then to read it out loud. Following this, the examiner asks a series of comprehension questions. Both the student's reading accuracy and reading comprehension are scored. A reading level (and corresponding age range) is determined if the student obtains > 95% correct in decoding and > 70% correct in comprehension.

2.7.2 Reading Success Project Assessments

In addition to the school-based measures, a number of assessments were conducted as part of the Reading Success project to monitor student progress over time, including response to interventions. This included the re-administration of key assessments described above including the YARC, the LeST, and the CC-2. Chapter 5 provides a description of the outcomes for the Year 4–5 cohort across these assessments following the relevant intervention programme.

2.8   Comparisons Between Project-Initiated Standardised Reading Assessments and School Reading Data

As described above, the school already implemented reading assessments as part of their common practice to monitor reading outcomes. As an additional reading assessment (i.e. the YARC) was administered as part of the Reading Success project, it was important to compare reading results on the YARC and these school-based measures. Comparing student performance across the tools allowed us to evaluate whether the school's existing reading assessments would accurately identify students who struggled in their reading comprehension and reading accuracy on the YARC. For this project, school-based data on the PM Benchmark and PAT-R collected at a similar point in time to the YARC were available. Chapter 3 reports these results.

2.9   Summary

This chapter provided an overview of the methodology that was used in the Reading Success project to (1) understand teacher perspectives around the teaching of reading, (2) identify students who show challenges in their reading accuracy and/or comprehension skills, and (3) evaluate student reading self-concept and motivation. It explained how the Simple View of Reading drives the reading assessment process and provided details of the theoretically based assessments that were used, including an overview of how to interpret different types of assessment results. Finally, the importance of ongoing monitoring of student performance was highlighted as students move from the learning to read to reading to learn phase.

Appendix 1: Pre- and Post-interview Prompt Questions

Pre-interview prompt questions

1. How would you describe your current school?
2. What is the general philosophy at this school?
3. What about the students who attend here?
4. Tell me about the programmes that are in place to support students' literacy learning.
5. Can you tell me about the students in the literacy support programmes?

6. What aspects of the school's philosophy and planning impact on these programmes?
7. What programmes are currently in place that aim to improve literacy outcomes for students?
8. What are the current perceptions of the success as well as areas in need of improvement of these programmes?
9. What future programmes and approaches to improving success in literacy learning might be considered in your school?

Post-interview prompt questions

1. Firstly, can you tell me how you were involved in the project?
2. What are your thoughts on how the project went?
3. What do you think worked well in this project?
4. What do you think could be improved?
5. Have you noticed any differences in your students? For example, more effective at reading, need more support?
6. What have you learnt from the project? For example, do you feel your skills related to the teaching of reading have improved? If so, how? And if not, why?
7. What do you think would help more in relation to the teaching of reading? And your students' reading skills?

Appendix 2: Sample of Assessment Tools to Complete the Speech-to-Print Profile

Spoken language assessments

Test details	Age range	Country where normed	Areas assessed + approx. administration times	Type of assessment	Comments	References
Underlying representations						
*Clinical Evaluation of Language Fundamentals—*5th Edition (CELF-5)	5; 0–21; 11	USA Australia	Spoken language; 30–45 min (core subtests)	Norm-referenced	• Includes *Understanding Spoken Paragraphs* subtest • Administered by: speech-language pathologists only	Wiig et al. (2017) (Aus version)
Test of Integrated Language and Literacy Skills (TILLS)	6; 0–18; 11	USA	Spoken (and written language); 90 min	Norm-referenced	• Includes language comprehension subtest • Administered by: speech-language pathologists, special educators, reading specialists, learning disability specialists, neuropsychologists, educational psychologists, and other educational specialists	Nelson et al. (2016)
*Peabody Picture Vocabulary Test—*5th Edition (PPVT-5)	2; 6–90; 0+	USA	Vocabulary knowledge (receptive); 10–15 min	Norm-referenced	• Administered by: allied health or special education professional	Dunn (2018)

(continued)

(continued)

Spoken language assessments

Test details	Age range	Country where normed	Areas assessed + approx. administration times	Type of assessment	Comments	References
Profile of Oral Narrative Ability (PONA)	4; 0–7; 6	Australia New Zealand	Narrative production and comprehension; 15 min	Local norms: Norm-referenced	• Administered by educators and speech pathologist • For instructions, go to: www.marleenwesterveld.com	Westerveld and Gillon (2010); Westerveld et al. (2012) Westerveld and Vidler (2016)
Test of Narrative Language—2nd Edition (TNL-2)	5; 0–15; 11	USA	Narrative production and comprehension; 15–20 min	Norm-referenced	• Not specified	Gillam and Pearson (2017)
Phonological processing						
Sutherland Phonological Awareness Test—Revised (SPAT-R)	YOS 1–4	Australia	Identification and manipulation of syllables, rhyme, and phonemes, and includes tests of non-word reading and spelling; 15 min	Norm-referenced	• Administered by: speech-language pathologists or education specialist	Neilson (2003)

(continued)

(continued)

Spoken language assessments

Test details	Age range	Country where normed	Areas assessed + approx. administration times	Type of assessment	Comments	References
Comprehensive Test of Phonological Processing—2nd Edition (CTOPP-2)	4; 0–24; 11	USA	Phonological processing Phonological memory Rapid automatic naming; 40 min	Norm-referenced	• Administered by: schools and speech-language pathologists	Wagner et al. (2013)
Lindamood Auditory Conceptualisation Test—Third Edition (LAC-3)	5; 0–18; 11	USA	Ability to perceive and conceptualise speech sounds; 20–30 min	Criterion-referenced	• Speech-language pathologists or occupational therapist	Lindamood and Lindamood (2004)
The Children's Test of Non-word Repetition	4; 0–8; 0	Britain	Assesses non-word repetition skills only; 15 min	Norm-referenced	• Not specified	Gathercole et al. (1994)
TILLS—non-word repetition subtest	As above	As above	Subtest assessing non-word repetition; 5–10 min	As above	As above	As above

(continued)

(continued)

Spoken language assessments

Test details	Age range	Country where normed	Areas assessed + approx. administration times	Type of assessment	Comments	References
Clinically Useful Words		Australia	Assesses multisyllabic word repetition skills only; 5 min	Informal	• Not specified	James (2006) Available from: https://speech-language-therapy.com/index.php?option=com_content&view=article&id=46
The Single-Word Test of Polysyllables	4; 0 +	Australia	Assesses multisyllabic word repetition skills only; 10–15 min	Informal	• Not specified	Gozzard et al. (2006)
Rapid Automatized Naming and Rapid Alternating Stimulus (RAN/RAS) Tests	5; 00-18; 11	USA	RAN—letters, numbers, colours, and objects RAS—letters and numbers; letters, numbers, and colours; 5–10 min	Norm-referenced	• Administered by: psychology, school counselling, occupational therapy, speech-language pathologists, social work, education, special education, or related field	Wolf and Denckla (2005)

Written language assessments

Test details	Age range	Country where normed	Areas assessed + approx. administration times	Type of assessment	Comments	References
Rule/concept knowledge						
Letter Identification Test	Not specified	Australia	Assesses letter identification knowledge; 5–10 min	Informal	No norms available	Available from: https://www.motif.org.au
Letter Sound Test	YOS K-3	Australia	Assesses sounding out single letters and letter combinations; 5–10 min	Norm-referenced		Available from: https://www.motif.org.au
Diagnostic Spelling Test—Sounds	YOS K-3	Australia	Assesses spelling of sounds using appropriate letters; 5–10 min	Norm-referenced		Available from: https://www.motif.org.au
Word level—word recognition						
Test of Word Reading Efficiency—2nd Edition (TOWRE 2)	6; 0–24; 11	USA	Real words and nonsense words; 10 min Individual	Norm-referenced	• Administered by: allied health or special education professional	Torgesen et al. (2012)

(continued)

(continued)

Written language assessments

Test details	Age range	Country where normed	Areas assessed + approx. administration times	Type of assessment	Comments	References
Castles and Colheart— 2nd Edition (CC2)	6; 0–11; 6	Australia	Regular, irregular, and nonsense words; 10 min	Norm-referenced		Available from: https://www.motif.org.au
Word level—spelling						
South Australian Spelling Test (SAST)	6; 0–15; 0	Australia	Assessment of single word spelling; 15–30min	Norm-referenced	Administered by: educators	Westwood (2005)
Test of Written Spelling—Fifth Edition	6; 0–18; 0	USA	Single word spelling; 20 min Group or individual	Norm-referenced	Allied health or special education professional	Larsen et al. (2013)
Diagnostic Spelling Test for Irregular Words	YOS 1–7	Australia	Spelling of irregular words; 10–30 min	Norm-referenced		Available from: https://www.motif.org.au
Diagnostic Spelling Test for Non-words	YOS 1–7	Australia	Non-word spelling; 10–30 min	Norm-referenced		Available from: https://www.motif.org.au

(continued)

(continued)

Written language assessments

Test details	Age range	Country where normed	Areas assessed + approx. administration times	Type of assessment	Comments	References
TILLS—non-word spelling test	As above	As above	Subtest assessing non-word spelling; 10 min	As above	As above	As above

Text level

Test details	Age range	Country where normed	Areas assessed + approx. administration times	Type of assessment	Comments	References
York Assessment of Reading for Comprehension (YARC)	5; 0–12; 0	• UK • Australia	Accuracy, rate, and comprehension; Individual 10–15 min	Norm-referenced	• Administered by: school psychologists, speech pathologists, and specialist teachers	Snowling et al. (2012)
Gray Oral Reading Test—5th Edition (GORT)	6; 0–23; 11	USA	Accuracy, rate, and comprehension; 20–30 min	Norm-referenced	• Administered by: allied health or special education professional	Wiederholt and Bryant (2012)

References

Australian Council for Educational Research. (2018). *Progressive achievement tests in reading (PAT-R).* Australia: Author.

Australian Curriculum Assessment and Reporting Authority [ACARA]. (n.d.). *ICSEA for principals.* Retrieved from https://www.myschool.edu.au/more-information/information-for-principals-and-teachers/icsea-for-principals/.

Australian Government. (2016). *National assessment program-literacy and numeracy (NAPLAN).* Retrieved from https://www.nap.edu.au/.

Barton, G. (2020). Recollage as tool for self-care: Reflecting multimodally on first five years in the academy through Schwab's lines of flight. *Qualitative Research Journal, 20*(1), 49–62. https://doi.org/10.1108/QRJ-04-2019-0039.

Barton, G., & McKay, L. (2014). *Impact report for Nerang state high school: A collaborative, community initiative.* Mt Gravatt: Griffith University.

Barton, G., & McKay, L. (2016a). Adolescent learners and reading: Exploring a collaborative, community approach. *Australian Journal of Language and Literacy, 39*(2), 162–175.

Barton, G., & McKay, L. (2016b). Conceptualising a literacy education model for junior secondary students: The spatial and reflective practices of an Australian school. *English in Australia, 51*(1), 37–45.

Bornholt, L. J. (2002). An analysis of children's task strategies for a test of reading comprehension. *Contemporary Educational Psychology, 27*(1), 80–98.

Bowyer-Crane, C., & Snowling, M. J. (2005). Assessing children's inference generation: What do tests of reading comprehension measure? *British Journal of Educational Psychology, 75,* 189–201.

Braun, V., & Clarke, V. (2006). Using thematic analysis in psychology. *Qualitative Research in Psychology, 3*(2), 77–101. https://doi.org/10.1191/1478088706qp063oa.

Cartwright, K. B., Marshall, T. R., & Wray, E. (2016). A longitudinal study of the role of reading motivation in primary students' reading comprehension: Implications for a less simple view of reading. *Reading Psychology, 37*(1), 55–91. https://doi.org/10.1080/02702711.2014.991481.

Castles, A., Coltheart, M., Larsen, L., Jones, P., Saunders, S., & McArthur, G. M. (2009). *Assessing the basic components of reading: A revision of the Castles and Coltheart test with new norms (CC2).* Retrieved from www.motif.org.au.

Chapman, J. W., & Tunmer, W. E. (1995). Development of young children's reading self-concepts: An examination of emerging subcomponents and their relationship with reading achievement. *Journal of Educational Psychology, 87*(1), 154–167. https://doi.org/10.1037//0022-0663.87.1.154.

Colenbrander, D., Nickels, L., & Kohnen, S. (2016). Similar but different: differences in comprehension diagnosis on the Neale Analysis of Reading Ability and the York Assessment of Reading for Comprehension. *Journal of Research in Reading.* https://doi.org/10.1111/1467-9817.12075.

Cunningham, A., & Carroll, J. (2011). Age and schooling effects on early literacy and phoneme awareness. *Journal of Experimental Child Psychology, 109*(2), 248–255. https://doi.org/10.1016/j.jecp.2010.12.005.

Dunn, D. M. (2018). *Peabody picture vocabulary test* (5th ed.). Minneapolis, MN: Pearson Assessments.

Gathercole, S., Willis, C., Baddeley, A., & Emslie, H. (1994). The children's test of nonword repetition: A test of phonological working memory. *Memory, 2,* 103–127.

Gillam, R., & Pearson, N. (2017). *Test of narrative language* (2nd ed.). Austin, TX: Pro-Ed.

Gozzard, H., Baker, E., & McCabe, P. (2006). Children's productions of polysyllabic words. *ACQuiring Knowledge in Speech, Language and Hearing, 8*(3), 113–116.

Heilmann, J., & Malone, T. O. (2014). The rules of the game: Properties of a database of expository language samples. *Language, Speech, and Hearing Services in Schools, 45*(4), 277–290.

James, D. G. H. (2006). *Hippopotamus is so hard to say: Children's acquisition of polysyllabic words (Doctoral thesis).* Sydney, Australia: University of Sydney.

Katzir, T., Lesaux, N. K., & Kim, Y.-S. (2009). The role of reading self-concept and home literacy practices in fourth grade reading comprehension. *Reading and Writing, 22*(3), 261–276. https://doi.org/10.1007/s11145-007-9112-8.

Keenan, J. M., & Betjemann, R. S. (2006). Comprehending the Gray oral reading test without reading it: Why comprehension tests should not include passage-independent items. *Scientific Studies of Reading, 10*(4), 363–380.

Keenan, J. M., Betjemann, R. S., & Olson, R. K. (2008). Reading comprehension tests vary in the skills they assess: Differential dependence on decoding and oral comprehension. *Scientific Studies of Reading, 12*(3), 281–300.

Lambert, S. D., & Loiselle, C. G. (2008). Combining individual interviews and focus groups to enhance data richness. *Journal of Advanced Nursing, 62*(2), 228–237.

Larsen, S., Hammill, D., & Moats, L. (2013). *Test of written spelling* (5th ed.). Austin, TX: Pro-Ed.

Larsen, L., Kohnen, S., Nickels, L., & McArthur, G. (2015). The Letter-Sound Test (LeST): a reliable and valid comprehensive measure of grapheme–phoneme knowledge. *Australian Journal of Learning Difficulties, 20*(2), 129–142. https://doi.org/10.1080/19404158.2015.1037323.

Leitch, S. (2006). *Prosperity for all in the global economy: World class skills. Final report of the Leitch review of skills.* London: The Stationery Office.

Liamputtong, P., & Rumbold, J. (2008). *Knowing differently: Arts-based and collaborative research methods.* New York: Nova Science Publishers.

Lindamood, P. C., & Lindamood, P. (2004). *Lindamood auditory conceptualization test-third edition.* Austin, TX: Pro-Ed.

McNiff, S. (2008). Art-based research. In J. G. Knowles & A. L. Cole (Eds.), *Handbook of the arts in qualitative research: Perspectives, methodologies, examples, and issues* (pp. 29–40). Thousand Oaks, CA: Sage.

Nation, K., & Snowling, M. (1997). Assessing reading difficulties: The validity and utility of current measures of reading skill. *British Journal of Educational Psychology, 67*, 359–370.

Neale, M. D. (1999). *Neale analysis of reading ability* (3rd ed.). Melbourne, VIC: Australian Council for Educational Research.

Neilson, R. (2003). *Sutherland phonological awareness test—revised (SPAT-R) Revised.* Jamberoo, NSW: Author.

Nelson, N. W., Plante, E., Helm-Estabrooks, N., & Hotz, G. (2016). *Test of integrated language and literacy skills (TILLS).* Baltimore, MD: Brookes.

Parkin, C., & Parkin, C. (2011). *PROBE 2: Reading comprehension assessment.* Wellington, NZ: Triune Initiatives.

Semel, E., Wiig, E. H., & Secord, W. A. (2006). *Clinical evaluation of language fundamentals—fourth edition—Australian* (Standardised ed.). Marrickville: Harcourt Assessment.

Smith, A., Nelley, E., & Croft, D. (2009). *PM Benchmark reading assessment resources (AU/NZ).* Melbourne: Cengage Learning Australia.

Snowling, M. J., Stothard, S. E., Clarke, P., Bowyer-Crane, C., Harrington, A., Truelove, E., & Hulme, C. (2012). *York assessment of reading for comprehension* (YARC), (Australian ed.). London: GL Assessment.

Torgesen, J. K., Wagner, R. K., & Rashotte, C. A. (2012). *Test of word reading efficiency* (2nd ed.). Austin, TX: Pro-Ed.

Wagner, R. K., Torgesen, J. K., & Rashotte, C. A. (2013). *The comprehensive test of phonological processing—second edition (CTOPP-2).* Austin, TX: Pro-ed.

Westerveld, M. (2009). Measuring reading comprehension ability in children: Factors influencing test performance. *ACQuiring Knowledge in Speech, Language and Hearing, 11*(2), 81–84.

Westerveld, M. F., & Gillon, G. T. (2010). Profiling oral narrative ability in young school-aged children. *International Journal of Speech-Language Pathology, 12*(3), 178–189. https://doi.org/10.3109/17549500903194125.

Westerveld, M. F., Gillon, G. T., & Boyd, L. (2012). Evaluating the clinical utility of the profile of oral narrative ability in 4-year-old children. *International Journal of Speech-Language Pathology, 14*(2), 130–140. https://doi.org/10.3109/17549507.2011.632025.

Westerveld, M. F., & Vidler, K. (2016). Spoken language samples of Australian children in conversation, narration and exposition. *International Journal of Speech-Language Pathology, 18*(3), 288–298. https://doi.org/10.3109/17549507.2016.1159332.

Westwood, P. (2005). *Spelling: Approaches to teaching and assessment* (2nd ed.). Melbourne: Australian Council for Educational Research.

Wiederholt, J. L., & Bryant, B. (2012). *Gray oral reading tests—fifth edition*. Austin, TX: Pro-Ed.

Wiig, E. H., Semel, E., & Secord, W. A. (2017). *Clinical evaluation of language fundamentals Australian and New Zealand* (5th ed.). Bloomington, MN: NCS Pearson.

Wolf, M., & Denckla, M. B. (2005). *RAN/RAS: Rapid automatized naming and rapid alternating stimulus tests*. Austin, TX: Pro-ed.

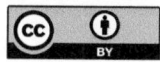

Part II
The Reading Success Project (Results)

Chapter 3
Reading Success Results Across the Year Groups

Rebecca M. Armstrong, Marleen F. Westerveld, and Georgina M. Barton

Abstract This chapter describes the Reading Success results across the year groups and compares the students' performance on the *York Assessment of Reading for Comprehension* (YARC) with results from school-based reading measures. For students in their *learning to read* phase (Year 1), we also report their Year 2 results. For students in their *reading to learn* phase of schooling (Year 4), we only report their reading results at the end of that school year. All results are described using our five-step assessment to intervention framework, based on the Simple View of Reading. We demonstrate how the assessment results can be used to create speech-to-print profiles for students who can be categorised as demonstrating: (a) specific word reading difficulties; (b) mixed reading difficulties; (c) specific comprehension difficulties; and (d) non-specified reading difficulties. Based on these profiles, we suggest which students may benefit from supplemental intervention (i.e. Tier 2 or Tier 3).

Keywords Reading assessment · Reading comprehension · Reading rate · Reading accuracy

3.1 Learning to Read Cohort Results

As described in Chap. 2, parental consent for their children's participation in the project was provided for 93 students attending Year 1. These students were seen in Term 4 of Year 1. The following sections first provide an overview of the results obtained through the five-step assessment to intervention process (see Fig. 2.2), with suggestions for supplemental intervention when indicated.

3.1.1 Step-by-Step Assessment Results—Year One

Step 1: Assess Reading Skills

All Year 1 students were assessed on the *York Assessment of Reading for Comprehension* (YARC; Snowling et al., 2012) in Term 4 of the school year. As a group,

© The Author(s) 2020
M. F. Westerveld et al., *Reading Success in the Primary Years*,
https://doi.org/10.1007/978-981-15-3492-8_3

these students in the *'learning to read'* phase of development scored within normal limits on the three YARC scales (see Table 3.1): reading accuracy (RA), reading rate (RR), and reading comprehension (RC). It should be noted that reading rate can only be calculated if students complete levels 1 and 2 of the YARC (as opposed to the beginner level and level 1).

Step 2: Further Assessment of Students who Scored below Expectations on RC

As shown in Table 3.1, when applying a standard score cut-off of 85, 26 students scored below expectations on the RC component of the YARC.

i.   We first checked if students' poor performance in RC could be explained by their challenges in RA. Only 6 of the 26 students demonstrated poor RA on the YARC.
ii. The next step was ascertaining the listening comprehension (LC) skills for the 26 students who scored below expectation in their RC ability. One student left the school between assessment points, and therefore LC data were only available for 25 students. It was found that 8 of these 25 students scored below expectations on the language comprehension task (*Understanding Spoken Paragraphs* subtest of the CELF-5; Wiig, Semel, & Secord, 2017).

After checking RA and LC skills, there were 16 students who demonstrated RC difficulties and performed within expectations for both LC and RA. Therefore, these students were classified as showing *non-specified reading difficulties*. Of these 16 students, 6 students demonstrated low RR (SS < 85), and 4 students had RR not calculated.

The flow chart in Fig. 3.1 provides a visual representation of the reading profiles for all students in Year 1, including the 26 students who performed below expectations for RC, including their skills in RA and LC.

Step 3: Further Assessment of Word Recognition Skills

Further assessments of the 6 students with poor RA were conducted. These results showed that 5 of the 6 students with RA scores below expectations also showed orthographic difficulties on the LeST (Larsen, Kohnen, Nickels, & McArthur, 2015), i.e.

Table 3.1 Student performance on the *York Assessment of Reading for Comprehension* ($n = 93$)

	Reading accuracy (RA) $n = 93$	Reading rate (RR) $n = 80$	Reading comprehension[a] (RC) $n = 92$[b]
Mean (SD)	101.47 (13.17)	95.27 (13.88)	93.78 (14.10)
Range	70–130	70–122	70–127
n (%) below SS80	4 (4.3%)	10 (10.8%)	14 (15.1%)
n (%) below SS85	8 (8.6%)	22 (23.7%)	26 (28%)

[a]There was no significant difference between reading comprehension scores based on gender ($p = 0.599$) or E/ALD ($p = 0.452$) when applying SS85 cut-off.; [b]1 student had poor RA on beginner level that meant RC was not able to be administered and therefore missing data

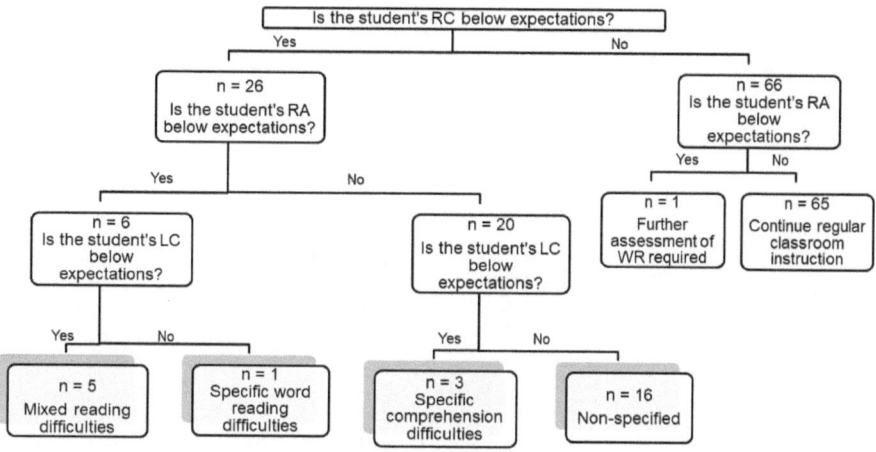

Fig. 3.1 Results from Steps 1 and 2 from the assessment to intervention process. One student had left the school by step 2

z-score < -1.0. Only 2 of the 6 students performed below expectations for phonological awareness (score below the 25th percentile) on the *Sutherland Phonological Awareness Test—Revised* (SPAT-R: Neilson, 2003). The single word reading assessment (CC-2; Castles, Coltheart, Larsen, Jones, Saunders, & McArthur 2009) showed strengths and difficulties across the 6 students, but all students performed below expectations on at least one word type (i.e. regular, irregular, and/or nonsense words).

Step 4: Creating Speech-to-Print Profiles ($n = 26$)

The assessment results for the 26 students who performed below expectations for RC were compiled to provide an overall picture of their strengths and weaknesses in the different domains assessed. The reading results for each reading profile for these 26 students are described below and shown in Tables 3.2, 3.3, 3.4, and 3.5.

Specific Word Reading Difficulties Only 1 student (S303) presented with a specific word reading difficulties (SWRD) profile. As shown in Table 3.2, this student showed difficulties in RA at both the text level and single word level. However, the student's RA difficulties did not seem to arise as a result of weaknesses in orthographic knowledge or PA skills.

Mixed Reading Difficulties Table 3.3 outlines the assessment results for the five students with mixed reading difficulties profiles at the end of Year 1. As shown, these students had difficulties with both RA and LC. Based on further assessment of their reading skills, it was also found that all 5 students demonstrated difficulties in single word reading, as well as orthographic knowledge. Only 2 (S40 and S17) of the 5 students showed difficulties with phonological awareness.

Given the challenges across WR and LC, we recommend that students with this type of profile receive supplemental intervention at a Tier 2 (or Tier 3) level of

Table 3.2 Assessment results for students with a specific word reading difficulties (SWRD) profile in Year 1

Code	Gender	E/ALD	RC SS	RA SS	RR SS	LC SS	Single word reading			Orthographic knowledge[a]	PA
							REG[a]	IR[a]	NW[a]		
S303	F	N	83	81	NC	10	−1.16	−1.37	−0.36	0.95	WNL

Note E/ALD English as an additional language or dialect; *RC SS* reading comprehension standard score; *RA SS* reading accuracy standard score; *RR SS* reading rate standard score; *LC SS* language comprehension scaled score; *PA* phonological awareness; *REG* regular words; *IR* irregular words; *NW* nonsense words; *NC* not calculated/completed; *WNL* within normal limits; [a]z-scores reported

Table 3.3 Assessment results for students with a mixed reading difficulties profile in Year 1

Code	Gender	E/ALD	RC SS	RA SS	RR SS	LC SS	Single word reading			OK[a]	PA
							REG[a]	IR[a]	NW[a]		
S190	M	N	70	79	70	4	−0.47	−1.26	−0.14	−1.2	WNL
S26	F	Y	<70	76	NC	6	−1.52	−2.03	−1.46	−1.2	WNL
S40	F	Y	<70	74	NC	6	−1.16	−1.65	−0.27	−2.41	BNL
S38	M	N	<70	84	NC	4	−1.22	−0.73	−1.03	−1.04	WNL
S17	M	N	<70	83	NC	4	−1.59	−1.37	−1.65	−1.75	BNL

Note E/ALD English as an additional language or dialect; *RC SS* reading comprehension standard score; *RA SS* reading accuracy standard score; *RR SS* reading rate standard score; *LC SS* language comprehension scaled score; *OK* orthographic knowledge; *PA* phonological awareness; *REG* regular words; *IR* irregular words; *NW* nonsense words; *NC* not calculated/completed; *WNL* within normal limits; *BNL* below normal limits; [a]z-scores reported

Table 3.4 Assessment results for students with a specific comprehension difficulties (SCD) profile in Year 1

Code	Gender	E/ALD	RC SS	RA SS	RR SS	LC SS
S93	M	N	< 70	88	NC	6
S95	M	N	75	86	75	6
SS0	M	Y	80	86	81	5

Note E/ALD English as an additional language or dialect; *RC SS* reading comprehension standard score; *RA SS* reading accuracy standard score; *RR SS* reading rate standard score; *LC SS* language comprehension scaled score; *NC* not calculated/completed

support, targeting both WR and LC skills based on their end-of-Year 1 performance. With improved WR, these students would still be at risk of specific comprehension difficulties (considering their poor performance in LC), and continued monitoring should be in place.

Specific Comprehension Difficulties Table 3.4 shows the assessment results for students identified with SCD. Because these students demonstrated adequate performance in RA at the text level (based on the YARC), no further testing of single word reading, orthographic knowledge, or PA was conducted. As shown in Table 3.4, the students with SCD profiles at the end of Year 1 showed specific difficulties in language comprehension, suggesting they would benefit from supplemental intervention targeting their LC and RC skills.

Non-specified Reading Difficulties Table 3.5 shows the results for students who could not be categorised into one of the three reading profiles described above. As shown in Table 3.5, 11 of these 16 students with NS reading difficulties profiles demonstrated challenges with RR (either SS < 85 or unable to be calculated). For these students, ongoing monitoring is suggested, and further testing may be required. For example, difficulties in RR could be indicative of phonological retrieval difficulties and these students may thus require further assessment in this area. However, there are other possible explanations for the poor RC performance of some of these students, resulting in a non-specified reading difficulties profile without clear challenges in WR or LC. We have listed possible reasons in the final column of Table 3.5 (see also Chap. 1 for more detail).

Poor Comprehension Monitoring To adequately respond to the questions following the reading of a passage, students need to monitor their comprehension while reading. One example is participant S16 who showed excellent reading accuracy (SS 117) as well as a very fast reading rate (SS 113). This rapid rate may have hindered this student's ability to monitor her comprehension; when administering a language comprehension task, S16 scored well within normal limits (SS10 on the *Understanding Spoken Paragraphs* subtest of the CELF-5).

Limited Capacity Working Memory Model (Crystal, 1987) Another consideration for the NS profiles is that these students are still in the 'learning to read' phase of development, which means that more cognitive resources are needed for decoding, with fewer cognitive resources available for RC, particularly for students whose reading rate is poor. These results suggest that ongoing monitoring for students

Table 3.5 Assessment results for Year 1 students with a non-specified reading difficulties profile

Code	Gender	E/ALD	RC SS	RA SS	RR SS	OK[a]	LC SS	Possible reasons for low RC
S27	M	Y	82	100	101		8	Comprehension monitoring
S48	F	N	80	107	98		8	Comprehension monitoring
S308	M	N	80	97	93		10	Comprehension monitoring
S92	F	N	74	107	87		8	Comprehension monitoring
S31	M	Y	84	90	87		9	Comprehension monitoring
S16	F	N	< 70	118	113		10	Comprehension monitoring
S22	M	Y	74	94	80		10	Poor reading fluency
S23	F	Y	< 70	90	NC		11	Poor reading fluency
S71	M	Y	80	100	80		10	Poor reading fluency
S49	F	N	< 70	86	NC	−1.8	8	Poor reading fluency—poor single word reading (regular)
S45	M	N	83	88	NC	−2.0	10	Poor reading fluency—poor single word reading
S37	F	N	83	85	NC	−1.4	9	Poor reading fluency—poor single word reading (regular and nonsense words)
S75	M	N	74	87	80	−1.0	7	Poor reading fluency—poor single word reading (and language borderline)
S30	F	N	72	89	77		12	Poor reading fluency—single word reading WNL

(continued)

Table 3.5 (continued)

Code	Gender	E/ALD	RC SS	RA SS	RR SS	OK[a]	LC SS	Possible reasons for low RC
S79	F	N	84	88	75		10	Poor reading fluency—single word reading WNL
S98	F	N	84	86	75		8	Poor reading fluency—single word reading WNL
S29	M	Y	83	88	NC		NA	

Note E/ALD English as an additional language or dialect; *RC SS* reading comprehension standard score; *RA SS* reading accuracy standard score; *RR SS* reading rate standard score; *OK* orthographic knowledge; *LC SS* language comprehension scaled score; *NC* not calculated/completed; *WNL* within normal limits; *NA* not available. [a]z-scores reported

with NS profiles may be required, and further assessment should be conducted if difficulties in any reading domains persist.

3.1.2   Considerations When Changing Assessment Cut-off to SS80

When conducting standardised assessments with normative data, it is important to consider changes to reading profiles when different cut-offs are used to determine reading performance. The decisions described in the previous sections were based on employing a 1SD cut-off to indicate reading performance that was 'below expectations'. As a result, we identified just over 28% of students needing follow-up assessment at the end of Year 1. However, according to the YARC manual, SS < 80 is used to indicate performance that is within the 'severe' range. If we had applied this SS80 cut-off in the Reading Success project, we would have identified 14 students with RC skills that were below expectations (i.e. 15%; see Table 3.1). Following the same assessment steps as described above and using a more stringent cut-off of SS < 80, we would have identified the following reading profiles: mixed reading difficulties profile: $n = 3$; specific word reading difficulties: $n = 0$; specific comprehension difficulties: $n = 4$; and non-specified: $n = 7$. It is important that the school team uses a collaborative approach in determining what cut-off will be applied to indicate reading performance and understands the potential implications. In this case, using a cut-off of SS80 may have been acceptable, although our research design does not allow us to draw definitive conclusions. Regardless, it is important to consider other available data, such as how the student is functioning in the classroom context to guide the interpretation of assessment results and help inform the intervention plan for each student.

3.1.3 Summary—Year One Experimental Test Results

The results for the 'learning to read' cohort show that when using the YARC as a standardised test of reading performance, using SS85 as a cut-off, approximately 28% of students were considered at risk, based on their RC performance in the learning to read phase of development. Using our step-by-step approach based on the SVR as a framework, four different reading profiles were identified at the end of Year 1. The students' performance on the YARC assessment was compared with the results from school-based reading measures (i.e. PM Benchmark Reading Assessments). We will discuss these results in the following section.

3.2 School-Based Versus Experimental Test Results—Learning to Read Cohort

During the early school years, the school used the PM Benchmark Reading Assessments (Smith, Nelly, & Croft, 2009; see Chap. 2). Based on this individually administered test, students were categorised as average or below average (using level 16 as the benchmark for satisfactory performance). In this section, we compare the students' performances on the assessments administered as part of the Reading Success project with the results from the PM Benchmark, a school-based reading measure.

3.2.1 Year 1: YARC RC Versus PM Benchmark

We found a significant moderate to strong correlation between student performance on the PM Benchmark (level) and their performance on the YARC RC (SS), $r = 0.68$ ($p < 0.001$). Table 3.6 shows the results comparing the students' performance on the YARC RC subtest (applying SS85 cut-off) and the PM Benchmark. As shown in Table 3.6, 75/92 students were correctly identified as performing within or below expectations (81.5%). However, 17/92 students were misidentified (18.5%); i.e. the results from one test did not match the results from the other test. These results are

Table 3.6 Year 1 students identified with reading difficulties on the RC component of the YARC versus the PM Benchmark

			PM Benchmark	
			Average	Below average
YARC RC	WNL		62 (67%)	4 (5%)
	Below expectations		13 (14%)	13 (14%)

Note PM PM Benchmark Reading Assessments; *YARC RC York Assessment of Reading for Comprehension, Reading Comprehension; WNL* within normal limits

Table 3.7 Reading data of the 13 Year 1 students who passed PM Benchmark but who performed below expectations on the YARC RC subtest

Code	Gender	E/ALD	PM	RC SS	RR SS	RA SS	USP	Reading profile
S30	F	N	21	72	77	89	12	NS
S37	F	N	16	83	NC	85	9	NS
S31	M	Y	21	84	87	90	9	NS
S48	F	Y	21	80	98	107	8	NS
S27	M	Y	24	82	101	100	8	NS
S22	M	Y	16	74	80	94	10	NS
S16	F	N	24	< 70	113	118	10	NS
S308	M	N	24	80	93	97	10	NS
S92	F	N	18	74	87	107	8	NS
S71	M	Y	17	80	80	100	10	NS
S29	M	Y	16	83	NC	88	NA	NA
S38	M	N	21	< 70	NC	84	4	Mixed
S20	M	Y	19	80	81	86	5	SCD

Note E/ALD English as an additional language or dialect; *PM* PM Benchmark Reading Assessment in level of achievement; *SS* standard score with 85–115 indicating performance within age expectations; *USP Understanding Spoken Paragraphs* subtest of the CELF-5; *NS* non-specified; *NC* not calculated; *NA* not available; *SCD* specific comprehension difficulties

discussed further below. It is important to note, however, that the PM level is based on a child's performance across decoding and comprehension skills, whereas the YARC reports a student's skills separately across these two domains. Thus, while the following compares these assessments in terms of identification of children at risk of reading difficulties, the differences across the assessments must be acknowledged and considered when interpreting these comparisons.

Table 3.7 outlines the assessment data for the 13 students who performed within average expectations for their year level on the PM Benchmark, but failed to meet expectations on the YARC RC component. As shown, 10 of these 13 students had profiles consistent with 'non-specified' reading difficulties at the end of Year 1.

As shown in Table 3.6, a further 4 students showed average RC skills on the YARC at the end of Year 1 but failed to meet the benchmark for PM. These students' results are shown in Table 3.8.

3.2.2   Year 1: YARC RA Versus PM Benchmark

Next, we compared performance on the RA component of the YARC with PM Benchmark performance. We found a strong correlation between student performance on

Table 3.8 Reading data of four Year 1 students who performed below expectations for PM Benchmark but who performed within normal limits on the YARC RC subtest

Code	Gender	E/ALD	PM	RC SS	RR SS	RA SS	Reading profile
S9	M	N	15	98	76	99	Typical
S87	M	Y	11	104	83	92	Typical
S299	M	N	14	86	87	89	Typical
S32	M	N	9	93	NC	81	Typical

Note E/ALD English as an additional language or dialect; *PM* PM Benchmark Reading Assessment in level of achievement; *RC* reading comprehension; *SS* standard score with 85–115 indicating performance within age expectations; *RR* reading rate; *RA* reading accuracy; *NC* not calculated

Table 3.9 Year 1 students identified with reading difficulties on the RA component of the YARC versus the PM Benchmark

		PM Benchmark	
		Average	Below average
YARC RA	WNL	74 (79%)	11 (12%)
	Below expectations	1 (1%)	7 (8%)

Note PM PM Benchmark Reading Assessments; *YARC RA* York Assessment for Reading Comprehension Reading Accuracy; *WNL* within normal limits

the PM Benchmark (level) and their performance on the YARC RA (SS), $r = 0.81$ ($p < 0.001$). The results from this comparison are shown in Table 3.9.

As shown in Table 3.9, 81 students met expectations on both assessments (87%). However, 12 students (13%) only met expectations on one of the tests. Only one student performed well on the PM Benchmark (level 21) but did not reach expectations in RA on the YARC (S38; see Table 3.7). This student showed a mixed reading difficulties profile. The breakdown of assessment results for the remaining 11 students who performed below expectations on the PM Benchmark but showed satisfactory performance in RA on the YARC is shown in Table 3.10. The three students with 'typical' Year 1 reading profiles based on the YARC RA (S9, S87, S299) in the table below are also included in Table 3.8 when investigating which students performed WNL on the YARC RC, but below expectations on the PM Benchmark.

3.2.3 Summary Year 1 YARC Versus PM Benchmark Results

Performance on the PM Benchmark was significantly correlated with student performance on the YARC RA ($r = 0.81$) and YARC RC ($r = 0.68$). Furthermore, use of the PM Benchmark resulted in correct classification of 81% of students who performed poorly in RC on the YARC. However, using the PM Benchmark does not differentiate between students' reading profiles and may miss some students who

Table 3.10 Reading data of 11 Year 1 students who performed below expectations on the PM Benchmark, but within expectations for RA on the YARC

Code	Gender	E/ALD	PM	RC SS	RR SS	RA SS	Reading profile
S9	M	N	15	98	76	99	Typical
S87	M	Y	11	104	83	92	Typical
S299	M	N	14	86	87	89	Typical
S93	M	N	7	70	NC	88	SCD
S95	F	N	12	75	75	86	SCD
S79	F	N	10	84	75	88	NS
S45	M	N	14	83	NC	88	NS
S98	F	N	15	84	75	86	NS
S75	M	N	13	74	80	87	NS
S49	F	N	7	70	NC	86	NS
S23	F	Y	11	70	NC	90	NS

Note E/ALD English as an additional language or dialect. *PM* PM Benchmark Reading Assessment in level of achievement. *RC* reading comprehension; *SS* standard score with 85–115 indicating performance within age expectations; *RR* reading rate; *RA* reading accuracy; *NC* not calculated; *SCD* specific comprehension difficulties; *NS* non-specified

show reading comprehension difficulties. Thus, if the PM Benchmark is being used within schools to assess reading performance, we recommend other available data (e.g. based on classroom performance) are also considered by school teams to supplement the PM Benchmark results and ensure students with reading comprehension difficulties are being correctly identified in the early years.

3.3 Follow-up Results One Year Later—Year Two

All students were closely monitored during Year 2 with some students obtaining supplemental intervention targeting their areas of difficulties (i.e. WR, LC, or both, depending on their reading profiles). Most of the students were reassessed for monitoring purposes in Term 4 of Year 2, and these results are discussed below.

A total of 70 students (75% of the original cohort of 93) were available (with parental consent) for follow-up assessments one year later (Year 2). Four students had left the school, and parent/caregiver consent forms were not returned for 19 students. Of these 19 students, five had been 'flagged' as at risk, based on their performance in RC (see Fig. 3.1). The results of the Year 2 YARC performances are displayed in Table 3.11.

When investigating these students' performance on the YARC in Year 1, the following results were found:

Table 3.11 Student performance on the *York Assessment of Reading for Comprehension* $(n = 70)$ in Year Two

	Reading accuracy $n = 70$	Reading rate $n = 68$	Reading comprehension $n = 70$
Mean (SD)	100.99 (12.2)	100.68 (14.1)	99.86 (13.1)
Range	75–130	70–124	73–130
n (%) below SS85	4 (5.7%)	10 (14.7%)	6 (8.6%)

- Of the 4 students (S40, S49, S17, and S45) who scored below SS85 in RA in Year 2, two students showed challenges in RA in Year 1 (S40 and S17), and all four had shown difficulties with reading rate as well as significant difficulties in orthographic knowledge (z-scores < -2.0).
- Of the 10 students who scored below SS85 in RR in Year 2, all 10 students had also shown challenges in RR in Year 1.
- Of the 6 students (S40, S23, S303, S82, S49, and S17) who scored below SS85 in RC in Year 2, five students showed challenges in RC in Year 1 (SS < 85) and 3 students showed challenges in RA in Year 1. All students except S82 had been flagged 'of concern' in Year 1. Unfortunately, no further assessment results are available for S82, as this student was away when we conducted our follow-up testing.

3.4 Overall Summary—Learning to Read Cohort

Using our five-step assessment to intervention framework, 28% of students at the end of Year 1 were identified as having reading difficulties. Using the SVR as a guide, four different reading profiles emerged. When comparing these results with school-based reading measures reasonably high correlations between the PM Benchmark data and student performance on the YARC RC and/or YARC RA were found with more than 80% agreement in classification of average versus below average readers on both assessments. Based on these results, the PM Benchmark may be a suitable reading assessment during the early years of schooling, although we recommend using a higher cut-off for the PM Benchmark and monitoring those students who end up on level 16 or 17, particularly for reading fluency. For example, teachers may administer the Test of Word Reading Efficiency 2nd Edition (TOWRE-2; Torgesen, Wagner, & Rashotte, 2012), which assesses a student's fluency in sight word reading and phonetic decoding skills and takes only 5 min.

When the students were reassessed one year later, many students showed a marked improvement. It was promising to see that at the end of Year 2 (third year of schooling), only 3 students showed significant reading difficulties; two of these students demonstrated a mixed reading difficulties profile (S40 and S17) and one (S49) showed

specific word recognition difficulties. These students require focused, more intensive support for WR. Further support is also indicated for all students who continued
to struggle in reading comprehension. Chapter 5 provides examples of interventions
that specifically target the language comprehension skills needed for successful reading comprehension. Finally, the importance of fluent decoding (as measured through
RR) should not be underestimated. Fluency in word recognition is needed to obtain
automaticity in reading skills to allow students to move from their learning to read
to reading to learn stage of schooling.

3.5 Reading to Learn Cohort Results

The five-step assessment to intervention process was also applied to students in
Year 4 (i.e. reading to learn phase of development). Parental consent for their children's participation in the project was provided for 78 students attending Year 4;
77 students were available for testing in Term 4 of Year 4. The following sections
provide an overview of the results from the five-step assessment to intervention process, with suggestions for supplemental intervention when indicated. Finally, the
students' reading performance on the YARC is compared to their results obtained
from school-based reading measures.

3.5.1 Step-by-Step Assessment Results—Year Four

Step 1: Assess Reading Skills

As a group, the students in the *reading to learn* phase of development (i.e. Year
4 cohort) scored within normal limits on the three YARC scales. These results are
shown in Table 3.12.

Table 3.12 Year 4 student performance on the *York Assessment of Reading for Comprehension* (n = 77)

	Reading accuracy n = 77	Reading rate n = 76	Reading comprehension[a] n = 77
Mean (SD)	91.97 (12.73)	88.18 (11.77)	88.26 (11.82)
Range	70–117	70–111	70–122
n (%) below SS80	15 (19.5%)	18 (23.7%)	23 (29.9%)
n (%) below SS85	23 (29.9%)	29 (38.2%)	33 (42.9%)

[a]There was no significant difference between reading comprehension scores based on gender ($\chi^2(1)$ = 0.070, p = 0.792) or E/ALD ($\chi^2(1)$ = 0.210, p = 0.647) using SS85 as cut-off

Step 2: Further Assessment of Students who Scored Below Expectations on RC

As shown in Table 3.12, 33 students scored below expectations on the RC component of the YARC.

i.   We first checked if students' poor performance in RC could be explained by their challenges in RA; 18 of the 33 students (54%) with poor RC demonstrated poor RA on the YARC.

ii. The next step was ascertaining the LC skills for the 33 students who scored below expectation in their RC. Only 32 of these 33 students were available for LC testing. It was found that 13 of the 32 students (41%) scored below expectations on the language comprehension task (*Understanding Spoken Paragraphs* subtest of the CELF-4; Semel, Wiig, & Secord, 2006).

After checking RA and LC skills, there were 9 students who demonstrated RC difficulties but performed within expectations for both LC and RA. Therefore, these students were classified as showing non-specified reading difficulties. Four of these students demonstrated low RR (SS < 85) on the YARC.

The flow chart in Fig. 3.2 provides a visual representation of the reading profiles for the 33 students who performed below expectations on RC, including their skills in WR and LC, and shows the reading profiles based on these assessment results.

Step 3: Further Assessment of Word Recognition Skills

Further assessments of single word reading were conducted with the 18 students with poor RA on the YARC. Of these 18 students with RA scores below expectations, a total of 17 showed difficulties in single word reading on the CC-2 across at least one

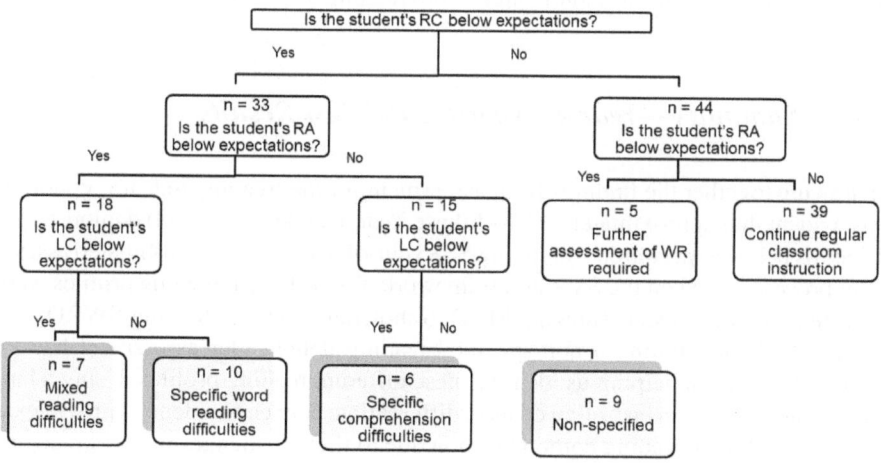

Fig. 3.2   Results from Steps 1 and 2 from the assessment to intervention process. One student was unavailable for testing at step 2

word type. Of interest, participant S09 performed below expectations in RA at the text level but demonstrated age-appropriate decoding skills across all single word types.

Step 4: Creating Speech-to-Print Profiles ($n = 33$)

The assessment results for the 33 students who performed below expectations for RC were compiled to provide an overall picture of their strengths and weaknesses in the different domains assessed. The reading results for these 33 students are shown in Tables 3.13, 3.14, 3.15, and 3.16.

Specific Word Reading Difficulties Ten students presented with a SWRD profile. As shown in Table 3.13, all students demonstrated weaknesses in RA at both the text level and single word level. Seven of these students also had underlying orthographic knowledge difficulties.

Mixed Reading Difficulties Table 3.14 outlines the assessment results for the seven students with MRD profiles. As shown, these students demonstrated difficulties with both RA and LC. Through further assessment of their reading skills, it was also shown that all students, except one, demonstrated difficulties in single word reading. These students should be considered for supplemental intervention at a Tier 2 or Tier 3 level of support, targeting both WR and LC skills.

Specific Comprehension Difficulties Table 3.15 presents the reading results for students identified with a specific comprehension difficulties profile. These students showed difficulties in comprehension, regardless of the modality (spoken or written).

Non-specified Reading Difficulties Finally, there were 9 students who performed poorly in RC, but showed adequate performance in RA (on the YARC) and on a language comprehension measure. The results are shown in Table 3.16. As previously described in Chap. 1, reasons for poor performance in RC could include difficulties in comprehension monitoring and working memory capacity (e.g. the students who showed difficulty with RR and/or single word reading, including S37, S23, and S41).

3.5.2 Summary—Year 4 Experimental Test Results

In drawing together the findings from assessment for the 'reading to learn' cohort, it was evident that approximately 43% of these Year 4 students ($n = 33$) demonstrated RC skills below expectations (applying SS85 cut-off). Using our step-by-step assessment process, based on the SVR as a framework, four different reading profiles were identified, with 7 students showing MRD, 6 showing SCD, 10 showing SWRD, and 9 students demonstrating a non-specified reading deficit. Our assessment battery seemed effective in helping us identify these different reading profiles. Using a language comprehension task allowed us to differentiate between students with dyslexia (who showed poor reading comprehension due to their challenges in word recognition) and those whose difficulties in language comprehension contributed to their low scores in reading comprehension. Further assessment of students who demonstrated

Table 3.13 Assessment results for students with specific word reading difficulties (SWRD) profiles in Year 4

Code	Gender	E/ALD	RC SS	RA SS	RR SS	LC SS	Single word reading			Orthographic knowledge[a]
							REG[a]	IR[a]	NW[a]	
S26[b]	M	Y	71	81	80	8	−1.53	−0.56	−2.35	−1.90
S46	M	Y	73	70	70	12	−2.48	−2.12	−2.62	−2.32
S51	F	N	75	78	70	7	−1.53	−0.76	−1.13	−1.51
S39	F	N	77	70	70	10	−2.29	−1.72	−1.57	−0.79
S59	M	Y	77	<70	75	7	−1.45	−1.37	−2.51	NC
S11[b]	F	N	77	83	80	11	−1.19	−1.35	−2.27	−0.68
S62	M	N	79	71	<70	7	−2.39	−1.37	−3.09	−2.34
S33[b]	F	N	79	74	<70	11	−1.96	−0.83	−2.83	−2.13
S43	M	N	81	83	82	11	−1.30	−0.91	−2.10	−1.80
S36[b]	F	N	83	78	80	10	−2.17	−0.91	−2.19	−1.13

Note E/ALD English as an additional language or dialect; *RC SS* reading comprehension standard score; *RA SS* reading rate standard score; *LC SS* language comprehension scaled score; *REG* regular words; *IR* irregular words; *NW* nonsense words; *NC* not completed; *WNL* within normal limits; *N/A* not available; [a]z-scores reported; [b]indicates these students received intervention as described in Chap. 5

Table 3.14 Assessment results for students with mixed reading difficulties profiles in Year 4

Code	Gender	E/ALD	RC SS	RA SS	RR SS	LC SS	Single word reading		
							REG[a]	IR[a]	NW[a]
S67	M	N	<70	<70	NC	3	−2.97	−3.09	−3.09
S66	F	N	<70	<70	<70	2	−2.30	−2.03	−3.09
S02	F	N	<70	71	<70	5	−2.31	−1.37	−2.42
S09	M	Y	70	83	99	3	0.12	−0.81	.33
S07	F	Y	73	77	<70	5	−1.85	−1.09	−2.10
S05	F	Y	77	71	85	3	−1.72	−0.76	−1.62
S61	F	N	84	83	80	6	−1.81	−1.25	−1.48

Note *E/ALD* English as an additional language or dialect; *RC SS* reading comprehension standard score; *RA SS* reading accuracy standard score; *RR SS* reading rate standard score; *LC SS* language comprehension scaled score; *REG* regular words; *IR* irregular words; *NW* nonsense words; *NC* not calculated/completed;
[a]z-score values reported

Table 3.15 Assessment results for students with specific comprehension difficulties (SCD) reading profiles in Year 4

Code	Gender	E/ALD	RC SS	RA SS	RR SS	LC SS	Single word reading		
							REG[a]	IR[a]	NW[a]
S68[b]	M	N	75	93	88	5	−0.22	−01.45	−0.87
S49[b]	F	N	75	93	90	6	−0.73	0.62	0.19
S74[b]	M	Y	83	95	77	3	−0.79	−1.35	−0.44
S56[b]	M	N	83	97	93	6	NC	NC	NC
S48[b]	M	N	83	85	94	5	−0.14	−0.21	−0.51
S31[b]	M	N	84	97	87	6	−0.73	−0.76	−0.13

Note E/ALD English as an additional language or dialect; *RC SS* reading comprehension standard score; *RA SS* reading rate standard score; *LC SS* language comprehension scaled score; *NC* not completed; [b] students participated in an intervention described in Chap. 5

Table 3.16 Assessment results for students with non-specified reading profiles in Year 4

Code	Gender	E/ALD	RC SS	RA SS	RR SS	LC SS	Single word reading		
							REG[a]	IR[a]	NW[a]
S37	M	N	81	85	75	10	−0.41	−1.77	−0.11
S71	F	N	77	97	93	8	NC	NC	NC
S60	F	Y	79	103	95	8	−0.73	−0.76	−0.38
S50	F	N	79	89	93	9	−0.73	0.41	−1.30
S17	F	N	73	91	77	10	−0.41	−0.21	−0.83
S57	M	Y	79	89	97	10	−0.14	−0.83	2.34
S23	M	N	73	91	82	11	−0.73	−1.09	−1.04
S65	F	N	84	95	87	8	NC	NC	NC
S41	M	N	79	93	82	12	−0.35	−1.09	−1.14

Note E/ALD English as an additional language or dialect; *RC SS* reading comprehension standard score; *RA SS* reading accuracy standard score; *RR SS* reading rate standard score; *LC SS* language comprehension scaled score; *REG* regular words; *IR* irregular words; *NW* non-words; *NC* not completed; [a] z-scores reported

poor performance in word recognition at text level (i.e. SWRD and MRD profiles) showed that all but one of these students demonstrated weaknesses in single word reading (non-word reading and regular word reading) using the CC-2; 70% of the students with SWRD showed significant difficulties with orthographic knowledge. Students' speech-to-print profiles may now be used to identify which skills should be targeted in intervention, whether it is at Tier 2 or Tier 3 within an RtI framework. A description of the interventions provided based on these reading profiles is described in detail in Chap. 5.

3.6 School-Based Versus Experimental Test Results—Reading to Learn Cohort

The students' performance on the YARC subtests was then compared to the data obtained as part of the school-based reading assessments. As described in Chap. 2, the PAT-R (Australian Council for Educational Research, 2018) was routinely used at the school to assess the reading skills of the Year 4 students. Data from 64 students were available.

3.6.1 Year 4: YARC Versus PAT-R

We compared students' performance on the PAT-R to their performance on the YARC RC and YARC RA subtests. Students were considered to score average on the PAT-R if their scaled score was ≥ 3; for the YARC subtests, we chose a cut-off of SS ≥ 85. We found significant, moderate correlations between performances on the PAT-R and the YARC RC ($r = 0.481$, $p < 0.001$) and between performances on the PAT-R and the YARC RA ($r = 0.487$, $p < 0.001$). Table 3.17 shows the results when cross-tabulating the students' scores.

Table 3.17 Year 4 ($n = 64$) students identified with reading difficulties on the RC component of the YARC versus the PAT-R

		PAT-R	
		Average	Below average
YARC RC	WNL	31	4
	Below expectations	12	17

Note PAT-R Progressive Achievement Tests in Reading; *YARC RC York Assessment for Reading Comprehension Reading Comprehension;* *WNL* within normal limits. Shading represents the students shown in Table 3.18

Based on these comparisons, 48 students (75%) were identified as either average or below average on both tests. However, performance on the two tests did not align for 16 students. Their results are shown in Table 3.18.

When comparing student performance on the YARC RA to their performance on the PAT-R, similar results were found (see Table 3.19). Based on these comparisons, 44 students (68%) were identified as either average or below average on both tests. However, performance on the two tests did not align for 20 students. Nine of the 20 students are included in Table 3.18; 4 students showed low reading accuracy on the YARC; 7 students showed poor reading comprehension.

Table 3.18 Performance of the 12 students who passed the PAT-R but performed below expectations on the YARC RC (shaded), as well as the 4 students who failed the PAT-R but performed WNL on the YARC RC

Code	Gender	E/ALD	PAT-R	RC SS	RA SS	RR SS	Reading profile
S07	F	Y	4	73	77	70	Mixed
S11	F	N	5	77	83	80	SWRD
S26	M	Y	4	71	81	80	SWRD
S33	F	N	4	79	74	70	SWRD
S36	F	N	4	83	78	80	SWRD
S40	F	N	5	83	72	77	NC
S48	M	N	6	83	85	94	SCD
S49	F	N	5	75	93	90	SCD
S50	F	N	4	79	89	93	NS
S56	M	N	5	83	97	93	SCD
S60	F	Y	7	79	103	95	NS
S65	F	N	4	84	95	87	NS
S04	F	N	2	85	91	71	Typical –low RR
S22	F	N	2	102	83	76	Typical – low RA/RR
S34	M	N	2	94	87	71	Typical – low RR
S69	F	N	2	90	101	94	Typical

Note Standard scores reported for the YARC; scaled scores reported for the PAT-R; *PAT-R* Progressive Achievement Tests in Reading; *RC* reading comprehension; *RA* reading accuracy; *RR* reading rate; *Mixed* mixed reading difficulties; *SWRD* specific word reading difficulties; *NC* non conclusive; *SCD* specific comprehension difficulties; *NS* non-specific reading difficulties

Table 3.19 Year 4 ($n = 64$) students identified with reading difficulties on the RA component of the YARC versus the PAT-R

		PAT-R	
		Average	Below average
YARC RA	WNL	33	10
	Below expectations	10	11

Note PAT-R Progressive Achievement Tests in Reading; *YARC RC* York Assessment for Reading Comprehension Reading Comprehension; *WNL* within normal limits

3.7 Overall Summary—Reading to Learn Cohort

Approximately 43% of the reading to learn cohort demonstrated poor reading skills at the end of Year 4 (i.e. their fifth year of schooling). In applying the five-step assessment to intervention process, four different reading profiles were identified. When comparing students' performance on the YARC RC and YARC RA with the PAT-R, between 68 and 75% agreement in classification of average versus below average readers was found. Closer inspection of the comparisons showed no clear pattern, although students with specific word recognition difficulties (dyslexia) were likely to perform well on the PAT-R. We suggest that the PAT-R may not be sensitive to reading challenges and recommend for the school to consider an alternative monitoring tool.

3.8 Chapter Summary

This chapter presented the results of the assessments conducted as part of the Reading Success project and described the comparisons between these assessment results and school-based data. Assessment results were reported for two distinct cohorts of children: (i) those in the learning to read phase and (ii) those in the reading to learn phase of development. It was shown that at the end of Year 1, 28% of the learning to read cohort demonstrated difficulties in RC. However, when these students were followed up 12 months later, only 9% showed persistent difficulties in RC at the end of Year 2, with the cohort showing improvements in all aspects of reading development. When considering the assessment results for the reading to learn cohort, approximately 43% of the students demonstrated poor RC skills at the end of Year 4. We showed that, when guided by the SVR as a framework, we identified which different underlying causes were contributing to the students' RC challenges, highlighting different reading profiles. Based on the findings reported in this chapter, we urge school teams to implement targeted interventions based on each student's reading profile. Finally, this chapter showed that while the PM Benchmark may be a suitable reading assessment during the early years of schooling, the PAT-R lacked sensitivity in detecting reading challenges in older readers.

References

Australian Council for Educational Research. (2018). *Progressive achievement tests in reading (PAT-R)*. Australia: Author.

Castles, A., Coltheart, M., Larsen, L., Jones, P., Saunders, S., & McArthur, G. M. (2009). Assessing the basic components of reading: A revision of the Castles and Coltheart test with new norms (CC2). Retrieved from www.motif.org.au.

Crystal, D. (1987). Towards a bucket theory of language disability: Taking account of interaction between linguistic levels. *Clinical Linguistics and Phonetics, 1,* 7–22.

Larsen, L., Kohnen, S., Nickels, L., & McArthur, G. (2015). The Letter-Sound Test (LeST): A reliable and valid comprehensive measure of grapheme–phoneme knowledge. *Australian Journal of Learning Difficulties, 20*(2), 129–142. https://doi.org/10.1080/19404158.2015.1037323.

Neilson, R. (2003). *Sutherland phonological awareness test—revised (SPAT-R)* (Revised ed.). Jamberoo, NSW: Author.

Semel, E., Wiig, E. H., & Secord, W. A. (2006). *Clinical evaluation of language fundamentals—fourth edition—Australian* (4th ed.). Marrickville: Harcourt Assessment.

Smith, A., Nelley, E., & Croft, D. (2009). *PM benchmark reading assessment resources (AU/NZ).* Melbourne: Cengage Learning Australia.

Snowling, M. J., Stothard, S. E., Clarke, P., Bowyer-Crane, C., Harrington, A., Truelove, E., & Hulme, C. (2012). *York assessment of reading for comprehension* (YARC), (Australian ed.). London: GL Assessment.

Torgesen, J. K., Wagner, R. K., & Rashotte, C. A. (2012). *Test of word reading efficiency 2 (TOWRE-2).* Austin, TX: Pro-Ed.

Wiig, E. H., Semel, E., & Secord, W. A. (2017). *Clinical evaluation of language fundamentals Australian and New Zealand* (5th ed.). Bloomington, MN: NCS Pearson.

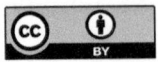

Chapter 4
Reading Self-Concept and Student Perceptions

Georgina M. Barton, Rebecca M. Armstrong, and Marleen F. Westerveld

Abstract This chapter describes the results of the Year 4 student responses to the *Reading Self-Concept Scale* (RSCS; Chapman & Tunmer, 1995). It then outlines three case studies that include data from interviews carried out with students involved in the programme. These students were selected on the basis of their low responses on the RSCS, regardless of their performance in reading. One member of the research team invited the students to participate firstly in a focus group where the students created a collage that represented themselves as a reader and also depicted how they felt about reading. The students were then invited to talk to the researcher in an individual interview with the collage as a stimulus for discussion and the development of strengths, weaknesses, opportunities, and threats chart. Findings showed that the students enjoyed reading for relaxation at home but felt the reading practices at school were not always as engaging as they could be for them. The chapter outlines a number of recommendations for schools and teachers in relation to the students' feedback.

Keywords Student perceptions · Reading self-concept · Reading ability · Primary school-age students

4.1 Introduction

As outlined in Chap. 1, it is important to investigate students' reading motivation. Previous research has suggested that motivation may show significant links with students' reading skills, both word recognition and comprehension (Cartwright, Marshall, & Wray, 2016). As explained by Cartwright et al. (2016), motivation may be influenced by students' expectations to do well on a task. In the Reading Success project, we investigated students' self-concept of reading, using the *Reading Self-Concept Scale* (RSCS) developed by Chapman and Tunmer (1995). This scale uses 30 items investigating: (a) perceptions of competence in reading, (b) perceptions of difficulty in reading, and (c) attitudes towards reading. Even though we were interested in describing the Year 4 cohort's self-perceptions, we wanted some more qualitative information from the students who rated themselves poorly on these scales. We interviewed three students, all of whom demonstrated the lowest scores on the RSCS,

© The Author(s) 2020
M. F. Westerveld et al., *Reading Success in the Primary Years*,
https://doi.org/10.1007/978-981-15-3492-8_4

regardless of their performance on a standardised reading test. The students' views and opinions expressed during the interviews were analysed to gain insight into their reading motivation. We explored these students' self-concept towards being a reader, but acknowledge that knowing more about the practices in their actual classrooms would assist in painting the full picture of their reading experiences. However, the aim of this book was not to describe or evaluate current literacy practices and we therefore did not systematically gather information on classroom literacy practices. Although results from the students' focus group and follow-up interviews provided more in-depth information, we acknowledge this was from the students' perspectives. Results from teacher interviews are reported in Chap. 7.

4.2 *Reading Self-Concept Scale*: **Group Performance**

All Year 4 students who participated in the Reading Success project were asked 30 questions from the RSCS (Chapman & Tunmer, 1995) to measure their reading self-concept. As shown in Table 4.1, overall, the students scored between 3 and 4 on all three subscales (on a scale from 1 [no, never] to 5 [yes, always] indicating generally positive perceptions regarding difficulty, competence, and attitude towards reading. These results are very similar to those reported by Chapman and Tunmer (1995). Closer inspection of individual student results showed that only 7 of the 78 students scored < 3 on the total RSCS. Ten students perceived reading to be difficult (scores < 3 for *difficulty*); 13 students perceived themselves as not very competent in reading (scores < 3 for *competence*); 8 students scored < 3 when asked about their *attitude* towards reading. We investigated correlations between subscales and found that the *difficulty* factor was correlated at $r = 0.67$ with *competence* ($p < 0.001$), $r = 0.26$ with *attitude* ($p = 0.023$) and $r = 0.80$ with total ($p < 0.001$); the *attitude* factor was correlated with *competence* at 0.40 ($p < 0.001$) and correlations between *attitude* and total scale was 0.86 ($p < 0.001$).

We also investigated the links between students' performance on the RSCS to their performance on the Reading Comprehension subtest from the *York Assessment of Reading for Comprehension* (YARC; Snowling et al., 2012). In our cohort of Year

Table 4.1 Year 4 performance on the *Reading Self-Concept Scale*		Whole sample $n =$ 77 M (SD)	RC below expectations $n = 33$ M (SD)	RC typical n = 44 M (SD)
	Difficulty	3.3 (.68)	3.0 (.69)	3.6 (.55)
	Competence	3.6 (.62)	3.4 (.64)	3.7 (.56)
	Attitude	4.2 (.67)	4.2 (.59)	4.1 (.73)
	Total	3.7 (.51)	3.5 (.52)	3.8 (.46)

Note RC Reading comprehension performance on the YARC

4 students, there was a positive, but mild correlation between reading comprehension and the total self-reported reading self-concept score ($r = 0.24$, $n = 77$, $p = 0.037$). This meant that students with higher RC scores also reported higher perceptions of their reading self-concept. When looking at the individual components of the RSCS, there was a statistically significant relationship between YARC RC score and self-perceptions in terms of *difficulty* ($r = 0.40$, $n = 77$, $p = < 0.001$). This can be interpreted to show that higher RC scores resulted in students' perceiving reading to be easier. However, there was no significant correlation between reading comprehension performance on the YARC and self-concept in terms of '*attitude*' towards reading ($r = 0.012$, $n = 77$, $p = 0.918$) and perceptions of *competence* in reading ($r = 0.143$, $n = 77$, $p = 0.215$). Finally, we considered the students' performance between subgroups of students who performed within expectations on the YARC RC (SS > 85) and those below expectations. As shown in Table 4.1, students who performed below expectations on the YARC RC (see also Chap. 3), found reading more *difficult* ($t(75) = -4.272$, $p = <0.001$), and perceived themselves as less *competent* ($t(75) = -2.609$, $p = 0.011$), but there were no group differences in *attitude* ($t(75) = .282$, $p = 0.779$) towards reading.

4.3 Student Interviews

To better understand the students' perceptions around reading and to gain insight into their reading experiences, a focus group was carried out with three students from Year 4 (pseudonyms: Daisy [S03], Lily [S33], and Tiana [S36]), who rated themselves the lowest on the *Reading Self-Concept Scale*. The students were invited to participate in a small group to create their own individual collage by using pre-cut images from magazines. The purpose of this activity was for the students to feel comfortable with the researcher initially in a small group. In the focus group, the main questions were (see also Chap. 2): (1) Tell me about you as a reader; and (2) Tell me about your experiences in reading. The students then returned individually at different times to talk to the researcher about their collage and themselves as a reader as well as reading in general. In this interview, a SWOT (strengths, weaknesses, opportunities, and threats) analysis was completed by each student where they talked about their own strengths and weaknesses as well as what would help and/or hinder their progress in reading. The questions used in each section of the SWOT analysis are shown in Table 4.2.

4.3.1 Results from the Focus Group

The students' focus group revealed a number of themes including enjoyment of reading, personal interest areas for reading, reading strategies, and reading groups at school. These themes are expanded below.

Table 4.2 SWOT questions for students

Strengths:	Weaknesses:
– What are you good at? At school? Outside of school? – What are you good at in terms of reading? – What about reading other types of texts, e.g. digital, multimodal, etc.? – What things do you like to learn about? – What do you know a lot about?	– What do you find difficult at school? – What are some things you would like to improve in your learning? – How do you think this improvement could happen? – What would help you? – Where/who do you currently get help from?
Opportunities:	Threats:
– Tell me about aspects of school that make you feel valued? Smart? – What about at home? – Who helps you with your learning? How often?	– What are some things that do not help you with learning? – What are the things you find most difficult?

Enjoyment and Topics of Reading

The students all stated that they liked reading. They all felt it helped them to relax and also provided an opportunity to not feel bored. Daisy liked to read with her sister. The students also shared their areas of interest in terms of the distinct topics and genres they liked to read.

> I like reading as you can just pick up a random book on any topic. It is relaxing. I also like reading because I can read if I get bored. I like reading about different cultures. I like reading French books. I am reading the book Chocolat with my mum. (Daisy)

> I like reading because you sometimes you feel like you just have to get away and sometimes it just takes you to a different world. I just like reading any type of book. I read magazines, newspapers, I like looking at the photos in the magazines, especially Kim Kardashian. (Lily)

> I like all sorts of books – the most I like is about plants and animals. (Tiana)

The students also talked about reading a wide range of text types including chapter books, magazines, information on their iPads, and non-fiction books such as about natural disasters.

Reading Strategies

The students spoke about what they did when they had challenges reading some of the texts they engaged in. Interestingly, from the three students, quite a number of different strategies were discussed including skipping words that are not familiar and seeing if the text still makes sense; using dictionaries; have an adult sound out difficult words; writing down the words and practising the spelling and finding out the meaning; asking for help.

> I like being a reader but sometimes I don't like reading cos there are really tricky words that I can't read and I don't understand and I can't sound out. I have trouble with really long words. (Lily)

I normally just skip the words but it makes sense to me. Mum says sound it out aloud but I don't like to do that because I am actually a really shy person. I had an incident where I read out aloud...(Daisy)

Reading Groups at School

Each student said that they were placed in a specific reading group at school. They explained that the reading groups were designed at different levels of proficiencies and included the red group, the green group, the pink group, and the blue group. Interestingly, although the reading groups changed once a term depending on student progress, the students all said that they had been in the same group all year despite them thinking they had probably improved enough to be moved up into the next group.

The students then completed their re-collages and attended an interview one at a time.

4.3.2 Interview Data Results

Results from Lily

Lily's (S33) performance on the *Reading Self-Concept Scale* indicated very low scores on ease of reading/difficulty and competence (1.8 and 2.2, respectively), but better on attitudes (3.6), indicating she perceived reading to be difficult and that she was not very confident, but maintained a positive attitude and liked reading. Lily's performance on the YARC showed significant difficulties in reading accuracy (SS 74) and reading rate (SS < 70), affecting her reading comprehension (SS 79). Her language comprehension was within normal limits (SS 11 on the *Understanding Spoken Paragraphs* subtest of the CELF-4; Semel, Wiig, & Secord, 2006). Lily demonstrated a *specific word reading difficulties* profile.

Lily talked about her collage (see Fig. 4.1) by saying she liked to read about animals, in particular dogs, and in cartoons. She also said she found reading relaxing, especially if she was reading outside and on the weekends. Lily liked to read chapter books and mentioned the Dork Diaries and books by author Paul Jennings. She talked about the reading groups in her classroom. These included the gold group—who needed more practise, silver group—who did not read bigger books, blue group—who had confidence, and turquoise group—who were more than average.

Lily described a range of strategies for reading in her interview. These included: read in her head, read aloud, sound out the words, guessing the meaning of the story, etc. She said her strengths as a reader related to being good at guessing or making inference and also reading in her head aloud.

Fig. 4.1 Lily's collage

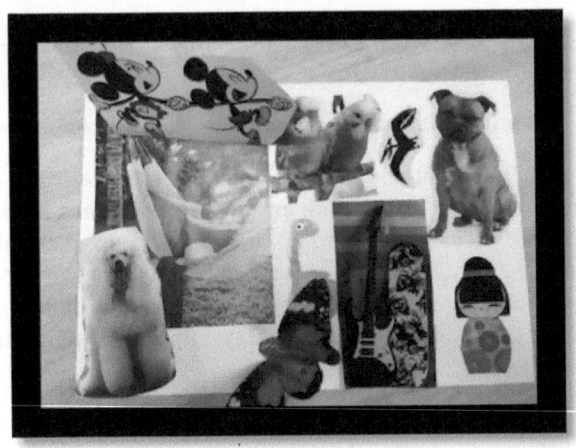

> Sounding out, reading a sentence and then come back to the word to try and figure it out myself because it's hard to understand some people when they put it in a way so I try to figure it out myself, and most of the time that helps because sometimes other people use these big words that I don't understand so I can help myself with it because I just don't understand other people what they say, so usually I help myself with it and if I don't I usually go to like my friends and if they can't help me I go to the teacher or my mum.

Lily mentioned that she mainly asks her mum for help as her dad is asleep a lot due to having to go to work at 3 am. She also said she is really busy with scouts and soccer, etc. Her dad also likes sports. This meant that most of her afternoons were busy with extra-curricular activities. Lily believed that her reading would improve through:

> Confidence in myself, so if I'm doing something, if I can just believe in myself and have courage…

> I could improve by looking at the pictures to help me figure out the words and asking for some help if I don't know…

She said she did not like to make mistakes as she was worried about other students' reactions.

Lily's SWOT is shown in Table 4.3 where the researcher noted down any comments Lily made but also observations.

Results from Daisy

Daisy's (S03) performance on the *Reading Self-Concept Scale* indicated very low scores on ease of reading/difficulty, competence, and attitude (1.9, 1.9, 2.9, respectively), indicating she perceived reading to be difficult, was not very confident, and had a reasonably low attitude towards reading. Daisy performed well on the YARC, with RC, RA, and RR all within normal limits. We did not receive Daisy's PAT-R results.

Table 4.3 Notes on Lily's SWOT

Strengths:	Weaknesses:
– Guessing the meaning of the text – Reading in her head not aloud – Sport: soccer, swimming, scouts, nippers – Maths	– Confidence in herself as a reader – Doesn't ask for help – Thinks she needs more reading strategies – To practise more – Speech, e.g. sounding out using coloured blocks – Spelling
Opportunities:	Threats:
– Ask for more help – Ask more questions – Use whisper phones—can hear themselves reading – Her mum is a reader – Her friends and teacher – She can rely on herself – More rotations—working with friends and reading aloud	– Doesn't like making mistakes – Worried about people bullying her for making mistakes – Needs to be quiet at home – Difficult to understand adults and their explanations – Never asked what she wants to learn or read

Daisy, in her interview, explained that her bedroom had just been renovated and they used pastel colours to create a relaxed feeling. As reading made her feel relaxed she chose images that used the same colour palette (see Fig. 4.2). The other items such as the cake, macrons, and the hanging chair all reminded her of how reading was relaxing and how she likes to read. The gems meant that she was achieving great things with her reading.

Daisy also talked about she was a dancer and is at dance 24/7. This experience influenced the types of books she read including ones with costumes. She also read about cooking and food as her mum had a Thermomix. Reading made her hungry, so she usually has snacks when she reads. She said reading made her feel relaxed

Fig. 4.2 Daisy's collage

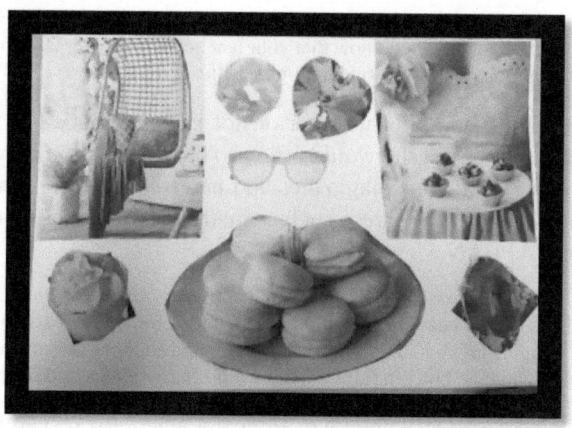

I like reading books about mysteries, like I like reading, like I've just finished this book about these girls went and lived in a palace and they kicked out because there was a special thing in the palace that they always wanted, they're like thieves cause they stole something in the palace, so they stole like a jewel from the palace, but there were two jewels that they wanted and so they had to keep going back and getting the jewels like without them getting kicked out…

I looked at it because it's kind of like a costume without the like tulle or whatever…and it's kind of like a costume and I like to read books about dance as well…at the moment I'm reading Chocolat and I, so me and my mum are reading that, and then by myself I'm reading the Maddie Diaries by Maddie Seigler which is really good and I like it.

In these comments, we can see that Daisy is able to recount the narratives from the books she was reading at the time.

At school, Daisy said she is part of the pink reading group, but she thinks she should be in the blue group. Her group had not changed throughout the entire year:

I think I've improved a lot with my reading, but like I would have liked to have moved up to the blue group but I don't know if I'm ready for that yet, like I can read really, like I've got the fluency, my teacher says I've got fluency, I've got expression, I've got like, I can connect to the text, she said I've got all that but I don't know if she thinks I'm ready to go up to the blue group…

I think because blue group is where all the really smart kids are…and they're really good readers so I don't think I'm up to their standards yet, I think I'm in the middle of their standards…

Daisy's comments showed that she was well aware of reading levels and what these levels entail. She could effectively gauge what type of reader she was and where she sat in relation to her peers. She was also aware of the areas of reading she found difficult and some strategies that could assist.

I think the words I find difficult because I'm only starting now to understand some words, like the words are a bit hard for me… Sometimes I have trouble understanding the meaning of the story…Unless I talk to mum about it… I don't understand the meaning of this story because a lot of the books I'm reading mum has read and I don't understand the meaning of the story.

I like getting criticism and feedback to help me grow because my mum said if you get criticism then you know that your teacher or whatever is, you know that you've got someone who is trying to help you do it so I like getting that.

When asked about whether or not Daisy felt she had a voice at school in terms of choice she said she would prefer to have the option of reading a wider variety of texts at school such as magazines and newspapers. She commented on feeling behind in her work in other areas such as maths, as the topics changed quickly particularly due to NAPLAN.

I try and ask for help, because I'm a year behind everyone, I can't keep up with the work as easy. I need, like usually we go on one topic, we learn that for a week and then the next topic, but I understand because we missed so much of our learning in NAPLAN and we have to do that, but I'm falling behind a bit in my maths and everything. (Daisy)

Daisy's SWOT is shown in Table 4.4 where the researcher noted down any comments Daisy made but also observations.

Table 4.4 Notes on Daisy's SWOT

Strengths:	Weaknesses:
– Reading recipes	– Her eyes sometimes don't work
– Reads a range of genres, e.g. French books, devices, diaries	– Maths
	– Decoding difficult words
– Reads outside for relaxation	– Summarising the meaning of texts
– Reading and oral expression fluency	– Can't provide honest feedback to peers or herself
– Has some metalanguage related to reading strategies	
– Finds feedback and information to assist	
Opportunities:	Threats:
– Her mum	– Doesn't like recording herself and listening
– Reading diversity and use of the library: she likes other countries, mysteries, and the Famous 5	– Lack of variety of text types; doesn't read magazines or picture books
	– Lack of reading in other curriculum areas
– Reading with her teacher	– Not asked what she wants to read in class but the higher levelled group is
– A family friend who helps at dance	
– That reading has to be interesting	

Results from Tiana

Tiana's (S36) performance on the *Reading Self-Concept Scale* indicated low scores for ease of reading/difficulty and competence, but relatively high scores for attitude (1.8, 2.2, 3.6, respectively). These scores indicate she perceived reading to be hard and was not very good at it. However, she liked reading and demonstrated a positive attitude towards reading. Tiana showed difficulties in reading accuracy and reading rate on the YARC (SS 78 and SS 80, respectively), which affected her reading comprehension (RC 83). She obtained a scaled score of 10 on the *Understanding Spoken Paragraphs* subtest of the CELF-4, indicating satisfactory performance in language comprehension. Tiana's single word reading (regular and non-words) was significantly affected (z-scores < -2.0). Tiana presented with a *specific word reading difficulties* profile.

Tiana's collage (see Fig. 4.3) included lots of images from the garden such as plants, flowers and a watering can. She explained that when she read she felt relaxed and it made her grow.

> I chose this because I like staying in the garden and I like reading in the garden. I always would like a big Japanese tree to read under. I like to talk to myself a lot because I am really lonely. I don't really have many friends. Reading makes me feel relaxed.

Such a metaphor was quite powerful for Tiana as reading for her at school was the opposite. In Year 1, she was asked to read aloud to the class but was very shy. When she did not say anything for about 30 s everyone laughed at her. This experience for Tiana impacted negatively on her reading confidence.

> The memories in Year 1 just keep coming back to me. When I read in a circle – I can't read out aloud – I don't like people hearing me. I like hiding behind someone. […] I didn't speak for 30 seconds and then everyone laughed at me. I am trying to get over it but it is really hard to get over it.

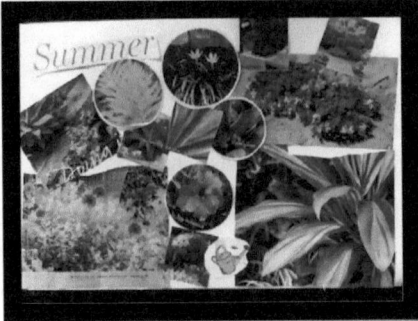 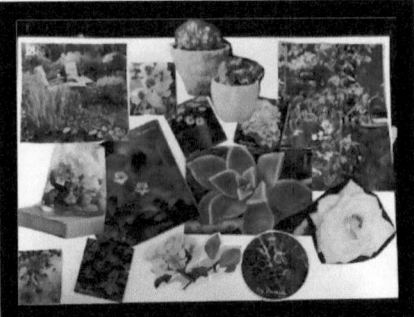

Fig. 4.3 Tiana's double-sided collage

Tiana talked about how she really did not like being singled out to read words or do spelling it made her feel 'really anxious'.

> I don't like people hearing me – even if you are in a corner. I get really anxious when it comes to spelling…I only like to do things when everyone does it I don't like being singled out. I like reading to our buddies.

In relation to meeting challenges with reading, Tiana talked about feeling frustrated sometimes but then she would usually find an easier book to read to feel better.

> Normally I feel like this with reading. Sometimes I just rage quit and get really angry and throw the book, I have some anger issues. Yeah I normally get a book that is easier to read. Like my dad's old yellow cat and dog book. It is about this friend who found a dog wandering in the forest. They make stuff together and talk together.

She also used a number of other strategies such as sounding out chunks of words that were difficult and ones she might experience when reading science texts.

> Sounding out chunks of the words and I use the strategy of seeing a word inside a word. I normally use that or if I have real trouble I skip the word and then come back to it so I know what it will mean…It is normally the long words. I really like science. Mum and dad said if you really like science we can go to a space place. There are really tricky words in science.

Tiana's SWOT is shown in Table 4.5 where the researcher noted down any comments Tiana made but also observations.

4.4   Discussion and Chapter Summary

As a group, the Year 4 students showed neutral to positive perceptions of their competence in reading. They perceived reading as not too difficult and demonstrated a positive attitude towards reading. These results are similar to those reported by Chapman and Tunmer (1995) almost 25 years ago. Closer inspection of the results from the current study showed that approximately 1 in 10 students demonstrated low

Table 4.5 Notes on Tiana's SWOT

Strengths:	Weaknesses:

– Science
– Letter chains—write the letters out for difficult words and sound out
– Tennis, handball
– Clarinet
– Taekwondo
– Readathon—read 40 books
   • Aussie Nibbles
   • Quests
	– Spelling—'rage quit'
	– Sounding words out in mind not aloud as too shy
	– Lack of confidence due to incident in Year 1 where class laughed at her
	– Maths—fractions
	– Needs to be in a group to learn—does not like being singled out

Opportunities:	Threats:
– Mum and dad – Using more of sounding out chunks of words – To find ways of becoming more confident – Practising writing – Partner reading – Reading to buddies out aloud	– Having to do oral presentations—gets very nervous – Hates being singled out—will hide from people – Fear of getting things wrong – Not saying words out aloud – Year 1 incident still a threat

reading self-concept, which may affect their reading motivation and hence hamper their reading performance. To better understand the views and perceptions of some of these students, we shared findings from three of the Year 4 students who participated in a focus group as well as individual interviews. They provided interesting feedback related to their self-perception as readers including the need to have choice in what they read, to receive support to improve their confidence towards reading, and to have the option of being able to change reading groups when possible. Generally, the students enjoyed reading outside of school but found reading practices in school stressful at times and often uninteresting. These findings are useful for teachers, the leadership team, and parents in relation to approaches to improving students' reading self-concept.

References

Cartwright, K. B., Marshall, T. R., & Wray, E. (2016). A longitudinal study of the role of reading motivation in primary students' reading comprehension: Implications for a less simple view of reading. *Reading Psychology, 37*(1), 55–91. https://doi.org/10.1080/02702711.2014.991481.

Chapman, J. W., & Tunmer, W. E. (1995). Development of young children's reading self-concepts: An examination of emerging subcomponents and their relationship with reading achievement. *Journal of Educational Psychology, 87*(1), 154–167. https://doi.org/10.1037//0022-0663.87.1.154.

Semel, E., Wiig, E. H., & Secord, W. A. (2006). *Clinical evaluation of language fundamentals—fourth edition—Australian* (4th ed.). Marrickville: Harcourt Assessment.

Snowling, M. J., Stothard, S. E., Clarke, P., Bowyer-Crane, C., Harrington, A., Truelove, E., & Hulme, C. (2012). *York assessment of reading for comprehension (YARC)*, (Australian ed.). London: GL Assessment.

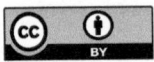

Chapter 5
Intervention Initiatives Across Three Levels of Instruction

Marleen F. Westerveld, Rebecca M. Armstrong, Georgina M. Barton, and Jennifer Peach

Abstract This chapter describes four evidence-based intervention initiatives at three levels of instruction (whole class, small group, and individual): (a) *Robust Vocabulary* Instruction was provided in Year 5 classrooms by the classroom teachers with support from the speech pathologist; (b) small-group intervention targeting expository structure was provided by the speech pathologist to Year 5 students demonstrating specific weaknesses in comprehension; (c) individual students participated in a specific training programme targeting orthographic knowledge, using a commercially available app, as well as phonological processing skills, using the LiPS programme; and (d) all foundation year classes participated in Read It Again—FoundationQ!, a supplementary whole-class oral language and emergent literacy intervention implemented by classroom teachers with coaching from the school-based speech pathologist. Results from all four intervention trials were positive and highlighted the importance of targeting specific areas of weaknesses in spoken or written language skills, based on the speech-to-print profile, to facilitate improvement in reading comprehension skills. Moreover, the importance of whole-class intervention during the learning to read stage was shown, with the cohort who received Read It Again performing better than the cohort who did not.

Keywords Intervention · Reading disorders · Phonological processing · Expository · Robust vocabulary

5.1 Robust Vocabulary Instruction

As outlined in Chap. 1, the importance of vocabulary knowledge to the reading process cannot be underestimated. Vocabulary knowledge during the preschool years is a strong predictor of future reading success (National Early Literacy Panel, 2008), and vocabulary knowledge during the school years has strong links with both word recognition and reading comprehension (Hiebert & Kami, 2005). For example, a student's ability to efficiently recognise words, particularly exception words such as 'yacht', is facilitated by their vocabulary knowledge (Dawson & Ricketts, 2017). Furthermore, students with better vocabulary skills perform better on tests of reading comprehension across the primary school years. Not surprisingly, the National

M. F. Westerveld et al., *Reading Success in the Primary Years*,
https://doi.org/10.1007/978-981-15-3492-8_5

Reading Panel (2000) stressed the importance of vocabulary instruction for reading success, and hence building teacher capacity in explicit and systematic vocabulary instruction contributes to a language-rich teaching and learning environment.

Research shows that the ability to acquire and express spoken vocabulary is a key to improve and sustain reading comprehension. The size of vocabulary, that is, the number and variety of words that students know, is a significant predictor of reading comprehension in the middle and secondary years of schooling, and of broader academic and vocational success (Beck, McKeown, & Kucan, 2013; Clarke, Truelove, Hulme, & Snowling, 2014). Students who lack adequate vocabulary have difficulty getting meaning from what they read. As a result, they may read less because they find reading difficult. Weak word recognition skills (including phonemic awareness, phonics, and fluency) also contribute to the gap between how much good and poor readers will read and encounter new vocabulary. As a result, they learn fewer words because they are not reading widely enough to encounter and learn new words.

Given this reciprocal relationship between reading and vocabulary growth, and the difficulties faced by struggling readers particularly relating to exposure, explicit instruction in vocabulary is considered one important intervention approach. Explicit or robust vocabulary teaching provides explanations of word meaning, across varied contexts, as well as multiple opportunities to explore and apply the words, which, in turn, can add substantially to the vocabulary growth of all students (Beck, McKeown, & Kucan, 2008). This teaching assists students to grow as readers and thinkers in both fiction and non-fiction, develops a deeper understanding of the words and concepts students are partially aware of, nurtures understanding of new concepts, increases reading comprehension, and enhances both oral and written communication skills (Allen, 1999). For this reason, Robust Vocabulary Instruction was conducted at the Tier 1 level of classroom support to facilitate vocabulary knowledge for all students.

5.1.1 Robust Vocabulary Instruction Overview

What it means to 'know' a word is not a simple notion. Word learning is *incremental*, that is, understanding a word is usually partial at first and grows with repeated exposures. Dale and O'Rourke (1986) conceptualised word learning as being along a continuum, ranging from never having seen or heard the word before, to having a deep knowledge of the word and its different meanings, and the ability to use the word confidently and accurately in speaking and writing contexts.

As outlined by Beck et al. (2013), research findings point to the need to create classrooms that support and encourage sophisticated word usage through a rich oral language environment characterised by:

- Multiple encounters (modelling and practice) in a variety of contexts;
- Rich and extensive opportunities to practise using new words that promote deep processing and more complex levels of understanding;

- Ample structured reviews to revisit learned words within and across lessons;
- Numerous opportunities to learn and reinforce vocabulary through wide independent reading;
- Nurturing an appreciation for words and how they are used; and
- Explicitly taught word meanings using clear, consistent, and understandable language.

The current project adopted the vocabulary instruction model proposed by Beck et al. (2013), in which vocabulary is classified into three tiers according to a word's frequency of use, complexity, and meaning. This classification of words into 'tiers' is based on the premise that not all words have equal importance when it comes to recommended instructional time.

Tier 1 words, or basic words, are words that usually develop without help, even if slowly. These words are seldom explicitly taught. Words such as 'dog', 'red', and 'big' would be classified as Tier 1 words, for example. Tier 2 words, or interesting words, are very important because of the role they play in literacy. Tier 2 words are the words that characterise written text—but are not so common in everyday conversation. What this means is that learners are less likely to be exposed to these words during everyday conversations. The opportunities to learn Tier 2 words come mainly from interaction with text. Because gaining meaning from written context is more difficult than gaining meaning from oral contexts, learners are less likely to learn Tier 2 words on their own in comparison with the words of everyday oral language. For example, words such as 'fortunate', 'ordinary', 'wonderful', and 'plead' would be classified as Tier 2 words. Tier 3 words are generally subject or domain-specific and as such do not have high use. These words are best learned if/when specific need arises. 'Isotope', 'conduit', and 'beaker' are examples of Tier 3 words.

In choosing words for instruction, McGregor and Duff (2015) suggested the following questions are asked:

- Is this word more likely to occur in written language than in spoken language?
- Would this word occur across various subject areas?
- Can the word be explained in student-friendly terms? A student-friendly explanation involves an explanation of a word's meaning in everyday, connected language.

Words selected for explicit instruction should be drawn from the curriculum; from texts or books read in class; or from assessment materials. The words targeted in the Reading Success project were Tier 2 words drawn from curriculum to the classroom (C2C) texts in conjunction with the speech pathologist and classroom teacher. These C2C materials included texts or books that would be read in class throughout the school term.

Intervention All school staff (across all year levels), including the leadership team, attended a 1-hour professional development (PD) session on Robust Vocabulary Instruction at the beginning of the school year. This PD covered the relationship between vocabulary and reading comprehension, Beck's tiers of vocabulary, word selection, student-friendly definitions, and the steps in Robust Vocabulary Instruction.

The Reading Success project then focused on Robust Vocabulary being implemented within the Year 5 cohort. As part of this project two Year 5 classrooms were 'control classes', meaning the teachers received the whole-school training at the beginning of the school year but chose to not actively complete the programme in their classrooms. The speech pathologist and the class teacher implemented Robust Vocabulary Instruction within two 'intervention classes' each week.

The intervention was provided at the whole-class level and included adhering to the nine steps for introducing a new word (see Appendix for a lesson plan *example*). Each week, six words were introduced. In the first four weeks, the speech pathologist introduced 3–4 words and the teacher observed. The teacher then completed the remaining 2–3 introductions and follow up for all words throughout the week, with one follow-up session being demonstrated by the speech pathologist. Follow-up activities aimed at providing the students with opportunities to: (1) use the Robust word in multiple contexts, (2) create links with other words, (3) use the Robust word in a sentence to show the meaning, and (4) ensure repeated exposure to the word. For example, the teacher may ask (1) the student to think of a person or job that relates to the word; (2) the teacher may ask the students to think of a word that has the opposite meaning; (3) the teacher provides an object or topic and asks the student to make a sentence related to the topic and containing the Robust word; and (4) the teacher may ask the student to describe the Robust word so that other students can guess what it is. For more examples of activities, please refer to the two books authored by Beck and colleagues (Beck et al., 2008, 2013). From week 5 onwards, the teachers were responsible for introducing all vocabulary words and completing the follow-up activities for the words during the week. To support fidelity of implementation across classrooms, an observation checklist was developed and completed by the speech pathologist in each classroom during the implementation of the programme.

Assessments All students participated in pre- and post-testing of 12 Tier 2 words, in the first week (week 1) and final week (week 10) of each school term. The words included in the testing comprised both Tier 2 words that would be targeted within the Robust Vocabulary Instruction that term (as described above) and also control words that would not be explicitly taught. The list of Tier 2 words that were included in the pre- and post-testing for Term 1 are shown in Table 5.1. Students were provided with a sheet of paper that included the target word, and space for writing their own definition of the target word and a sentence containing that word. Students were then given the following instructions:

Please write your name at the top of the sheet.

I will read each word and then I would like you to write what you think the word means in the first box. The meaning could be just one word that means the same as the word I read, or it could be a few words that explain the meaning. I would then like you to write a sentence that uses the word. (read example).This is not a spelling test and it doesn't matter if you spell words incorrectly in your sentences. Just have a go. If I read the next word and you haven't finished your sentence, you can come back to it later. You might not know some of these words, so I would just like you to do your best and have a go.

Table 5.1 The list of 12 Tier 2 words that were used for pre- and post-assessment

No	Word	Meaning	Sentence
Ex.	Delighted	Very happy	I was delighted when my mum bought my favourite cake for my birthday
1	Reliable		
2	Guarantee		
3	Diversity		
4	Attitude		
5	Genuine		
6	Raucous		
7	Imposing		
8	Colony		
9	Dwellers		
10	Menace		
11	Prevent		
12	Vulnerable		

Table 5.2 Score guide for robust vocabulary pre- and post-assessments

Points	Description	Relation to robust vocabulary instruction
0	Not able to provide a sentence or definition that reflects the meaning of the word	Never heard it before Heard it, but don't know what it means
1	Can provide a sentence that demonstrates some knowledge of the word. Has some difficulties defining the word	In context, I know it has something to do with…
2	Can provide a sentence and definition which reflects the true meaning of the word	Know it and use it

Student responses for each of the 12 words were scored from 0 to 2 according to the procedure outlined in Table 5.2. A total pre- and post-test score was then tallied for each student.

5.1.2 Intervention Results

Pre-and post-assessment results were available for 70 students, 36 of whom attended the intervention classes, and 34 attended the control classes. As explained above, each student was asked to provide the meaning for 12 words (six target words that were explicitly taught and six control words that were not explicitly taught) and provide a sentence that contains that word. Each response was scored on a scale of 0–2, which

Table 5.3 Group performance on target and control words prior to and the following intervention

	Target words		Pre-post	Control words		Pre-post
	Pre	Post	Effect size	Pre	Post	Effect size
Intervention classes	3.53 (2.0) 0–9	6.85 (2.4) 1–12	2.023*	3.18 (2.1) 0–8	4.1 (2.1) 0–8	0.582*
Control classes	3.47 (1.7) 0–7	4.61 (1.8) 1–7	0.753*	3.0 (1.4) 1–7	3.25 (1.8) 0–8	0.190

Note Max score is 12. * significant improvement in performance from pre to post ($p < 0.05$)

means the maximum score for this task was 24 (12 for the target words and 12 for the control words). Table 5.3 provides an overview of the results. To determine if the differences between the two groups were clinically significant, i.e. observable in the classroom, effect sizes were calculated and reported using Cohen's d (Cohen, 1988). Following Cohen's guidelines, $d = 0.2$ is considered a 'small' effect size, 0.5 represents a 'medium' effect size, and 0.8 represents a 'large' effect size. As shown in Table 5.3, although both groups showed a significant improvement on the target words following the school term, the intervention classes showed a much larger improvement, with a very large effect size. Only the intervention classes showed a significant improvement on the control words, with a large effect size.

5.1.3 Discussion

The results from this small-scale investigation showed that a Robust Vocabulary Approach, using an integrated service delivery model where speech pathologists and teachers work collaboratively to support vocabulary instruction was effective in enhancing student performance on a vocabulary task in which students were asked to demonstrate their understanding of Tier 2 words. Not only did the students in the intervention classrooms show better performance than their peers in the control classes on the target words post-intervention, they also demonstrated better performance on the control words. These results suggest that robust vocabulary may indeed 'kindle a lifelong fascination with words' (Beck et al., 2013).

5.2 Orthographic Knowledge and Phonological Processing Instruction

Based on the students' performance on the YARC reading accuracy subtest (Snowling et al., 2012), as outlined in Chap. 2 (step 3), combined with their performance on tasks tapping the skills needed for efficient word recognition skills, 12 students from the Year 4 cohort were invited to participate in an intervention programme aimed at enhancing orthographic knowledge as well as phonological processing skills. These students all demonstrated specific word recognition difficulties, as shown by the YARC reading accuracy, standard score < 85, accompanied by significant word reading difficulties on the CC-2 (Castles, Coltheart, Larsen, Jones, Saunders, & McArthur, 2009; motif.org.au), and low scores on the letter-sound knowledge test (LeST; Larsen, Kohnen, Nickels, & McArthur, 2015; motif.org.au). All students performed within normal limits in reading comprehension (SS $\geq$ 85 on the YARC) and/or language comprehension (SS $\geq$ 7 on the CELF-4, *Understanding Spoken Paragraphs*). These 12 students were then randomly allocated to an intervention or a control group, so that the intervention group received the intervention first, while the control group continued with their usual classroom instruction. As shown in Table 5.4 there were no significant group differences prior to intervention on any of the pre-intervention measures (all p's > 0.301). At this stage, we administered an additional measure of phonological processing, the *Lindamood Auditory Conceptualisation Test* (LAC;

Table 5.4 Student performance prior to the intervention

	LeST RS (/51)	Single word reading CC-2 (z-scores)			York Assessment of Reading for Comprehension (YARC)			CELF-4
		Reg	Irreg	NW	RA SS (AE)	RR SS	RC SS (AE)	USP (SS)
Intervention								
S22	38	−1.09	−1.37	−1.04	83 (7;11)	76	98 (9:10)	13
S26	31	−1.53	−0.56	−2.35	81 (7;11)	80	71 (6;11)	12
S33	29	−1.96	−0.83	−2.83	74 (7;9)	<70	79 (8;0)	11
S39	38	−2.29	−1.72	−1.57	<70 (6;5)	<70	77 (7;5)	10
S43	32	−1.30	−0.91	−2.1	83 (7;11)	82	81 (7;8)	11
S62	24	−2.39	−1.37	−3.09	71 (6;10)	<70	79 (7;5)	7
Mean	**32**	**−1.76**	**−1.13**	**−2.16**	**77**	**74.7**	**80.8**	**10.67**
Control								
S11	39	−1.19	−1.35	−2.27	83 (8;5)	80	77 (7;8)	11
S36	36	−2.17	−0.91	−2.19	78 (7;9)	80	83 (8;0)	10
S40	24	−1.77	−1.08	−2.23	72 (7;7)	77	83 (8;5)	10
S45	40	−1.28	−0.83	−1.43	74 (7;7)	83	122 (12;8)	11
S46	26	−2.48	−2.12	−2.62	<70 (6;4)	<70	73 (6;11)	8
S51	35	−1.53	−0.76	−1.77	78 (7;9)	70	75 (7;3)	7
Mean	**33.3**	**−1.74**	**−1.18**	**−2.09**	**75.8**	**76.7**	**85.5**	**9.5**

Note LeST Letter-Sound Test Raw Score (max 51); *CC-2* Castles and Coltheart; *CELF-4 Clinical Evaluation of Language Fundamentals*—4th Edition; *Reg* regular words, *Irreg* irregular words; *NW* non-words; *RA SS* Reading accuracy standard score; *RR* reading rate; *RC* reading comprehension (with age equivalent); *USP Understanding Spoken Paragraphs* (scaled score)

Lindamood & Lindamood, 2004), which measures the student's ability to discriminate speech sounds (phonemes) and to analyse the number and order of sounds in spoken patterns. Students are asked to demonstrate their knowledge by matching the number and the colour of small blocks to the number and patterns of sounds (e.g. show me /d//d/: two blocks, same colour; show me /m//ch//ch/, three blocks, first block a different colour to the next two blocks). According to the LAC manual, at the start of Year 5, the minimum recommended score is 86. All students scored below the minimum recommended score. There were no differences in performance between the intervention and the control group.

5.2.1   Intervention Overview

Students completed a six-week programme, comprising two sessions per week, one 30-mins individual session, and one 60-mins group (three students) session. Each session covered two components: (1) phonological processing and (2) orthographic knowledge. Although all students completed similar activities (as described below), the specific phonemes or phoneme combinations that were targeted in both components of the intervention were based on the students' performance on the LeST. The two components of the intervention will now be discussed in more detail below.

Phonological processing This programme explicitly targets students' phonological processing skills and was firmly based on Gillon and Dodd's (1995) work, in which ten students with significant reading difficulties participated. The programme itself is based on the Lindamood Phoneme Sequencing Programme, now into its fourth edition (LiPS; Lindamood & Lindamood, 2011), which systematically teaches students to segment, manipulate, and blend the speech sounds (phonemes) in syllables and words. We used Gillon and Dodd's adapted version of this programme by using traditional letter names to teach the students to encode sounds in syllables (using simple syllable sets, simple syllable chains, and complex syllables). We used the metalinguistic approach recommended in the LiPS programme which drew the students' attention to changes in syllables by explicitly describing these during the activities. The sessions involved reading and writing (of real and nonsense words) to ensure a transfer of segmentation and blending skills to reading and writing. Finally, as per the process outlined in the LiPS manual, the sessions included the teaching of some basic spelling rules (magic /e/; the /c/ in reading; two vowels go walking). Figure 5.1 provides an overview of the six-week programme.

Progress tracking sheets were used to monitor progress and to ensure students only moved on to the next level (simple syllables, CVC, varied, shifts) when they achieved 70–80% success at a certain level. Once a student was proficient with the coloured blocks, i.e. could quickly and accurately work through all levels using the coloured blocks and described the changes that were made with confidence, the student would only work with letter tiles. Use of progress checking sheets allowed for an individualised approach.

Week	Activities
Week 1	1. Tracking speech sound changes – coloured blocks, simple syllables (VC and CV). 2. Tracking speech sound changes – letter tiles, simple syllables. 3. Writing and reading simple syllables (game).
Week 2	1. Tracking speech sound changes with blocks, move from VC to C, to CVC and Varied. 2. Tracking speech sound changes with letter tiles as above. 3. Writing and reading simple syllables (game).
Week 3	1. Tracking speech sound changes with blocks, varied syllables, using a timer. 2. Tracking speech sound changes with letter tiles – aiming for 80% accuracy on CVC before moving to CCVC. 3. Writing and reading CVC words (game).
Week 4	1. Tracking speech sound changes with blocks, some students move on to shifts (e.g. *ask* to *aks*). Use a timer. 2. Tracking speech sound changes with letter tiles, using individualised tracking sheets to match students' orthographic knowledge. 3. Real word reading (CVC) – cut out and put face up on the desk. Read as many as you can in 1 min. 4. Real word and non word (CVC) spelling – write on cards. 5. Teach the magic /e/ rule: write the pairs on cards (e.g. *bit – bite*). 6. Board / bingo game – using the cards.
Week 5	1. Tracking speech sounds with blocks (only those students who had not yet achieved this level). Use a timer. 2. Tracking speech sound changes with tiles. 3. Real word reading in 1 min (using cards). 4. Simple spelling (CVC) – write on cards. 5. Teach the 'C in Reading' rule – write on cards. 6. Reading the cards (game).
Week 6	1. Tracking speech sound changes with blocks – improve your time. 2. Tracking speech sound changes with letter tiles – improve your time. 3. Real word reading (include magic /e/ and soft /c/ rules). 4. Teach the two vowels go walking rule – create cards. 5. Game – read the cards.

Fig. 5.1 Overview of the six-week programme targeting phonological processing skills

Orthographic knowledge Students' orthographic knowledge was targeted using the commercially available Reading Doctor App Letter Sounds 2 Pro (www. readingdoctor.com). The programme includes 70 of the most common letters-sound patterns and suffixes but was customised for each student based on their LeST results. The students were given access to the App twice a week for approximately 10–15 min, under supervision of the speech pathologist. As outlined on the Reading Doctor website:

Children are taught meaningful associations between the way that letters look and the speech sounds they typically represent through a unique system of visual, auditory and articulatory (speech sound) memory aids, or mnemonics. The teaching system in the app automatically identifies what a child knows, what the child does not know, and which letter sound patterns the child confuses. Letter Sounds™ 2 Pro teaches children to discriminate between confusing patterns, and strengthens weaknesses in letter-sound understanding.

Table 5.5 Mean group performance before and after intervention (SD in brackets)

Measures		Intervention group		Control group	
		Pre	Post	Pre	Post
Orthographic knowledge	LeST – raw scores	32 (5.4)	46.3 (3.7)	33.3 (6.7)	34.8 (7.8)
Single word reading CC-2	Regular words Raw score	24.7 (6.9)	28.5 (6.5)	24.8 (7.5)	25.3 (7.6)
	Irregular words Raw score	16.8 (2.6)	17.8 (1.7)	17.2 (3.2)	19.2 (5.3)
	Nonwords Raw score	7.0 (8.5)	18.2 (9.36)#	10.5 (6.7)	13.3 (5.8)
Reading Accuracy	YARC – RA SS	77.0 (6.0)	78.3 (4.2)	75.8 (4.8)	74.8 (7.3)

Note Shading indicates significant progress from pre- to post-intervention $p < 0.05$; # $n = 5$ as missing non-word data for B39

5.2.2 Intervention Results

All students were re-assessed after the six weeks of intervention on measures of orthographic knowledge (LeST), single word reading (CC-2), and reading accuracy (YARC RA). Repeated measures t-tests were used to calculate changes in performance from pre- to post-intervention. As shown in Table 5.5, the students in the intervention group demonstrated significantly greater gains ($p < 0.05$) on measures of letter-sound knowledge and single word reading (regular and non-words). No significant group differences were found on measures of irregular word reading or reading accuracy.

To determine if the differences between the two groups were clinically significant, i.e. observable in the classroom, effect sizes were calculated and reported using Cohen's d (Cohen, 1988). Following Cohen's guidelines, $d = 0.2$ is considered a 'small' effect size, 0.5 represents a 'medium' effect size, and 0.8 represents a 'large' effect size. As shown in Fig. 5.2, although both groups demonstrated progress over time, the intervention group made significantly more progress than the intervention group on measures of orthographic knowledge, regular, and non-word reading.

5.2.3 Discussion

The six-week intervention programme was effective in boosting students' performance in important print-related skills that underlie successful word recognition, i.e. orthographic knowledge and decoding of regular and nonsense words. Unfortunately, no generalisation was observed to the students' reading accuracy performance on the YARC. The most reasonable explanation is that the students need more time to apply their skills to sentence-level reading, which was not addressed in the intervention itself (i.e. the focus was on single words). Moreover, although most of the students

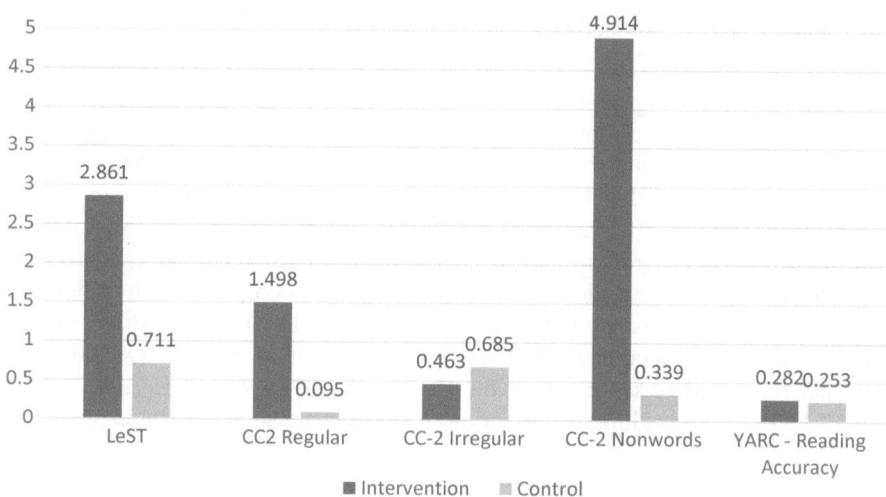

Fig. 5.2 Effect size comparison (Cohen's d) of the progress made in the intervention versus control group following six weeks of intervention

had made significant progress in single word reading (improving more than 1 z-score), closer inspection showed that many of the students still scored significantly below expectations (i.e. z-score < -1).

These results raise important questions regarding the timing of the intervention (Year 5). Research suggests intervention targeting word recognition difficulties is more effective during the earlier school grades than during the later years (see Wanzek & Vaughn, 2007). Early detection of reading difficulties is possible as long as sensitive and specific assessment tasks are used (see Chap. 3). By using an RtI approach, students showing early signs of dyslexia (i.e. fail to make satisfactory progress in word recognition despite high-quality classroom instruction) can then receive timely intervention. Another important issue to consider is the duration of the intervention. Although little is known about the exact dosage needed to effect more significant changes in reading accuracy, research suggests more extensive intervention is needed than the six weeks we provided as part of the Reading Success project (see Al Otaiba, Gillespie Rouse, & Baker, 2018). Finally, it is not clear what the active ingredients were as the intervention contained a combination of phonological processing and orthographic knowledge tasks, using both examiner- and computer-assisted instructional methods.

5.3   Expository Text Structure Intervention

Based on the students' performance on the YARC reading comprehension subtest (Snowling et al., 2012), followed by investigation of their reading accuracy performance on the YARC, and their performance on the *Understanding Spoken Paragraphs* subtest of the CELF-4 (Semel, Wiig, & Secord, 2006), as outlined in Chap. 2 (steps 1 and 2), eight students from the Year 4 cohort were invited to participate in an intervention programme aimed at enhancing their expository text structure knowledge. Six of these students demonstrated specific comprehension difficulties, as shown by the discrepancy between performance on the YARC reading comprehension and reading accuracy subtests (standard scores) accompanied by poor performance (i.e. standard score < 7) on the *Understanding Spoken Paragraphs* subtest of the CELF-4. The reading results for these students are shown in Table 5.6.

5.3.1   Intervention Overview

Students completed a six-week programme focusing on oral language in an expository context. The programme was adapted from Clarke, Snowling, Truelove, and Hulme (2010), who used a randomised control study design to investigate the effectiveness of three interventions aimed at improving the reading comprehension performance of 8- to 9-year-old students with specific reading comprehension deficits: text comprehension training, oral language training, and both trainings combined. All students received 30 h of intervention over 20 weeks (three 30-min sessions per week; two in pairs, one individually) implemented by a trained research assistant. Results from Clarke et al.'s (2010) study showed that the oral language groups made the greatest gains in reading comprehension following intervention. We adapted the intervention in the following ways:

- Duration and dosage. The intervention lasted six weeks (two 60-mins group sessions per week) for a total of 12 h of intervention per student. All sessions were in groups of four.
- Agent. The intervention was delivered by the speech pathologist.
- Focus. Our focus was on expository text, as opposed to narrative.

Similar to the Clarke et al. (2010) study, all sessions contained a range of evidence-based techniques, including "comprehension monitoring, cooperative learning, graphic organizers for story structure training, question answering and generating, summarisation, and multiple-strategy teaching" (p. 1108). Each session had the same structure and contained the four components of vocabulary, graphic organiser, reciprocal teaching, (figurative language, if applicable), and spoken expository (see Table 5.7). All sessions adhered to the following principles: (a) rich interaction and high-quality contextualised discussion; (b) integrate opportunities for relating material to personal experiences, and (c) exploration of vocabulary and spoken expository

Table 5.6 Student performance prior to (end of Year 4) and following the intervention (mid Year 5)

Groups	Age	Pre-YARC			CELF-4	Post-YARC		CELF-4	YARC	
		RA SS	RC SS	RC AE	USP (SS)	RC SS	RC AE	USP (SS)	RC AE pre-post	RC SS pre-post
Intervention										
S31	9;03	97	84	7;10	6	79	7;08	3		
S74	10;03	95	83	8;03	3	101	11;01	7		
S49	9;09	93	75	7;01	6	96	10;0	7		
S57	10;03	89	79	7;10	10	88	9;03	12		
Mean (SD)			80.3 (4.1)	7;11 (0;06)	6.25	91.0 (9.6)	9;06 (1;04)		p = 0.08 g = 1.27	p = 0.163 g = 1.06
Control										
S68	10;03	93	75	7;05	5	<70	7;01	3		
S56	9;11	97	83	7;10	6	85	8;09	5		
S48	10;03	85	83	8;03	5	74	7;08	10		
S23	9;06	91	73	6;08	11	<70	5;07	11		
Mean (SD)			78.5 (5.3)	7;07 (0;08)		74.8 (7.1)	7;04 (1;02)		p = 0.65 g = 0.138	p = 0.200 g = 0.43

Note YARC York Assessment of Reading for Comprehension, reading accuracy (RA), reading comprehension (RC); *USP Understanding Spoken Paragraphs* from the *Clinical Evaluation of Language Fundamentals* (CELF-4); *SS* standard score; *AE* age equivalence; g = Hegde's g

Table 5.7 Session overview of expository language intervention programme (adapted from Clarke et al., 2010)

Duration			
3 min	Introduction	Summary	Session 2
5 min	Vocabulary	Introduce a Tier 2 word, related to the topic, using a Robust Vocabulary Approach (Beck et al., 2013). Learning additional words through context	Session 2. Ask students to come up with a synonym and a sentence to demonstrate understanding
10 min	Graphic organiser	Introduce the passage article, or YouTube clip. Explain the type of expository it is and explain why	Repeat
10 min	Reciprocal teaching	Listen to the expository passage and write down keywords on the graphic organiser. Students raise their hand if they do not understand a concept, sentence, or passage. Model this behaviour Question generation activity: what, when, how, where, who, why, can, which? Activate background knowledge and develop visual representations; use reciprocal teaching strategies	Keywords or key phrases only Use a game with students drawing question cards they need to answer
5 min	Figurative language	If applicable. Explore non-literal language such as jokes, riddles, and idioms	Repeat
10–20 min	Spoken expository	Using the graphic organiser, one student provides oral summary; others provide feedback. Scaffolded by the SLP Practice is key	Students take turns and provide each other with feedback. Students are given a graphic organiser each with a pencil so they can tick if the other student has included the concepts/descriptors
3 min	Plenary	Wrap-up. Today we looked at…	

through varied games and activities, as well as worksheets. For further details see also Clarke et al. (2014).

The following five types of expository discourse were targeted during the intervention: (1) description, (2) procedure sequence, (3) comparison, (4) cause and effect, and (5) problem and solution. Each type of discourse had an accompanying graphic organiser, which was printed on A3 paper and used during the session. Graphic organisers were sourced online, for example, by performing a Google search or by visiting the www.readwritethink.org website. All five types of expository discourse were briefly introduced during the first session, and students were informed they would focus on a different type each week. The topic or content of the expository passages was matched to the topics that were covered in the classroom during those six weeks. For example, Unit 3.1 focused on '*the Riddle of the Black Panther–The Search*' (Education Services Australia). As a consequence, the first expository session focused on the Black Panther (*What's a Black Panther, Really?* National Geographic, 2015). Other sessions included comparing rugby union to soccer, why native goannas are dying (invaders), and flying foxes.

In week 6, the content of the previous five weeks was covered by introducing a topic (in this case 'flying foxes') and asking students what type of expository they could think of for the same topic, using the graphic organisers as prompts.

5.3.2 Intervention Results

All students were re-assessed after the intervention on Form A of the YARC to investigate their reading comprehension performance (standard score and age equivalence). Repeated measures t-tests were used to calculate changes in performance from pre- (i.e. at the end of Year 4) to post-intervention. As shown in Table 5.6, the students in the intervention group demonstrated larger gains in reading comprehension than the control group who participated in the regular classroom activities, as shown by the effect size (Hegde's g, whereby small effect [cannot be discerned by the naked eye] $= 0.2$; medium effect $= 0.5$; large effect [can be seen by the naked eye] $= 0.8$). Although the progress in reading comprehension made by the intervention group was not statistically significant ($p > 0.05$), the intervention group's performance showed a large effect size for both their standard score and their age equivalence (i.e. > 1 standard deviation change) compared to the control group who showed < 0.4 standard deviation change. These results indicate the experiment was underpowered (very small sample size), but also suggest the students in the intervention group made noticeable gains in reading comprehension following the intervention.

5.3.3 Discussion

The results from this pilot study showed the potential effectiveness of a short intensive intervention aimed at enhancing students' expository structure knowledge. Although replication is needed with larger numbers, our results are in line with those from previous studies (e.g. Clarke et al., 2010).

5.4 Supplementary Whole-Class Oral Language and Emergent Literacy Intervention

In response to the high literacy needs of the middle year students, the school implemented a supplementary whole-class oral language and emergent literacy intervention in the foundation year of schooling. This programme was based on Read It Again-PreK (Justice & McGinty, 2010), which is freely available online (see reference list), but adapted, with permission for the local context. The adapted version is called Read It Again—*FoundationQ*! (Department of Education, Training and Employment, 2013), and can be downloaded for free from the same website (see reference list).

5.4.1 Intervention Overview

Read it Again—*Foundation Q!* is a scientifically based oral language programme designed to develop and strengthen student's early foundations in four key areas of language and literacy—vocabulary, narrative, phonological awareness, and print knowledge:

> Read It Again - FoundationQ! is designed to systematically build students' language and literacy abilities in four areas. The scope of instruction encompasses: • Vocabulary - receptive and expressive repertoire of words • Narrative - ability to understand and produce extended discourse that describes real or fictional events occurring in the past, the present, or the future P a g e | 4 Read It Again – FoundationQ! • Phonological awareness - sensitivity to the phonological - or sound - structure of language • Print knowledge - interest in print, knowledge of the names and distinctive features of various print units (e.g. alphabet letters, words), and the way in which different prints may be combined in written language. (Department of Education, 2013, p. 3)

Read It Again is firmly based on current research regarding how adults can support children's language and literacy development using systematic and explicit instruction presented in highly meaningful literacy events such as storybook reading. A key feature of Read It Again is the repeated use of children's storybooks as a way to enhance language and literacy development. Studies indicate that repeated book reading influences both story-related vocabulary and story-related comprehension and that the average effect size for the relationship between repeated book reading and outcomes is larger when a book is read four or more times (Trivette, Simkus, Dunst, & Hamby, 2012; Zucker, Cabell, Justice, Pentimonti, & Kaderavek, 2013).

FoundationQ! is aligned to the Australian curriculum for the foundation (first) year of schooling and can be delivered as either a Tier 1 (differentiated) or Tier 2 (focused) teaching strategy within a response-to-intervention model. In this project, *FoundationQ!* was delivered as a Tier 1 strategy across all Prep (foundation year of schooling) classrooms. As explained in Chap. 1, differentiating instruction is a critical feature of a response-to-intervention model and advocates for active planning for student differences to ensure that every student is engaged, participating, and learning successfully (Goddard, Goddard, & Tschannen-Moran, 2007; Tomlinson, 2000).

Read It Again—*FoundationQ!* incorporates six differentiation strategies (three *Too Easy* strategies and three *Too Hard* strategies) that educators can use to scaffold students' performance on similar tasks or activities. To enhance teachers' use of the differentiated instructional strategies, a capacity-building model including coaching by the speech pathologist was implemented. The provision of coaching by speech pathologists is a natural extension of their consultative and collaborative services within a response-to-intervention framework and has been found to be effective when combined with in-service workshops (Milburn, Weitzman, Greenburg, & Girolametto, 2014). The professional development programme implemented employed a combination of a 1.5 h workshop that explained the intent, content, and structure of the programme and provided opportunities to identify and apply the *Too Easy* and *Too Hard* differentiation strategies; and individual coaching sessions incorporating demonstration lessons, scheduled observations, and instructional feedback.

To increase teachers' awareness of individual student needs and to assist teachers in differentiating instruction, Read It Again—*FoundationQ!* includes a student progress checklist (see the website for a copy), which measures individual students' progress against the learning objectives in each of the four domains specific to *FoundationQ!*. The checklists are administered at three separate points (after week 2, week 12, and week 21) during the 30-week intervention period. Development of skills is rated by teachers as:

- *Acquiring*: student never or occasionally demonstrates the skill
- *Building*: student often demonstrates the skill, but is not yet consistent and/or requires assistance, or
- *Competent*: student consistently demonstrates the skill

5.4.2 Intervention Results

To obtain preliminary data regarding the effectiveness of the implementation of this Tier 1 intervention initiative in reducing the overall number of students requiring additional support in oral and written language, we compared the performance of the

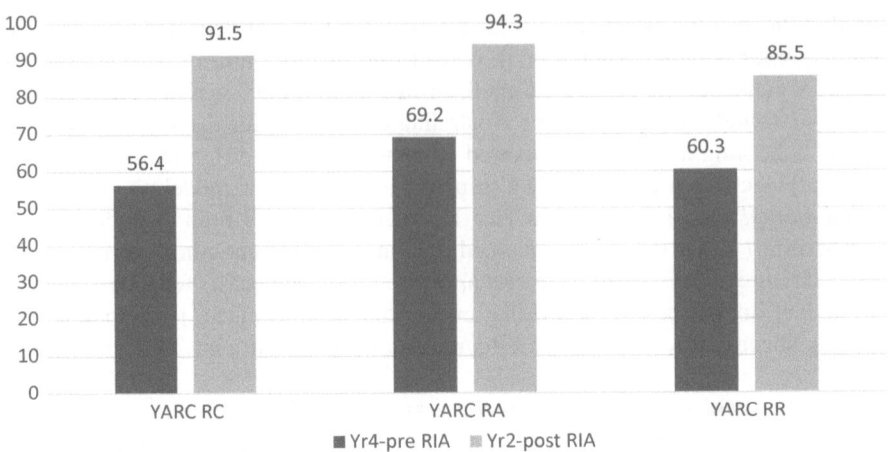

Fig. 5.3 Cohort (Year 2 vs. Year 4) performance on the YARC pre-and post-implementation of Read It Again (RIA): percentage of students performing within normal limits in reading comprehension, reading accuracy, and reading rate

Year 4 cohort ($n = 78$) who had not participated in the Read It Again—*FoundationQ!* programme (see Chap. 3 for specific cohort results) to the performance of the Year 2 cohort ($n = 69$; see Chap. 3 for specific cohort results when these students were in Year 1) on the YARC. On paper, these cohorts were similar with the Year 4 cohort comprising 6% indigenous students; 31% English as a Second Language (School ICSEA score 1005) and the Year 2 cohort comprising 6% indigenous students, and 35% ESL (ICSEA, 2013).

As shown in Fig. 5.3, a significantly higher percentage of students in Year 2 performed within normal limits (i.e. SS ≥ 85) on the YARC reading comprehension (91.5% vs. 57.1%). Similar results were seen for reading accuracy and reading rate.

5.4.3 *Discussion*

Implementation of Read It Again—*FoundationQ!* seems to be successful in lifting the literacy success rates of students attending the school. These findings provide preliminary evidence of the effectiveness of implementing this programme that was developed in the US (McGinty & Justice, 2010) but adapted for the Australian context, in Australian classrooms (see also Lennox, Westerveld, & Trembath, 2018). Further research is now needed to determine the effectiveness of these types of interventions for children with lower oral language ability (see Gillon et al., 2019).

5.5   Chapter Summary

This chapter presented the results from four evidence-based intervention initiatives. In the reading to learn cohort, Robust Vocabulary Instruction was provided at the whole-class level, with results showing larger gains in vocabulary knowledge in the intervention classes compared to the control classes. The other two intervention initiatives for this cohort of students involved students who had been identified with specific areas of weaknesses in spoken and/or written language skills impacting their reading comprehension performance. Expository structure intervention was provided to a group of students with specific comprehension difficulties, whereas a group of students with specific word recognition difficulties participated in an orthographic knowledge and phonological processing intervention programme. Results from these interventions were positive but modest, highlighting the importance of early identification of reading difficulties to enable more timely intervention. In the learning to read cohort, Read It Again—*FoundationQ*! was implemented at whole-school level in all Prep classes. Although our research design did not allow for firm conclusions regarding the effectiveness of this initiative, cohort mapping results showed a significant improvement in reading performance over time prior to and following the implementation of Read It Again—*FoundationQ* within the school. Implementation of the five-step assessment framework introduced in this book will now be needed to identify those students who need additional support, as our previous research has shown that implementation of this type of whole-class supplementary oral language and emergent literacy intervention alone may not be sufficient for long-term reading success (Lathouras, Westerveld, & Trembath, 2019).

Appendix Example of Lesson Plan Outlining the Nine Steps to Introducing a New Word

Introduction to word Tier 2 Target: misconception	
Steps of introduction	Tier 2 target word outline
1. Text or Activity Teacher reads the text to the students or completes other Key Learning Area activity	Text: **'What's a Black Panther, Really?'** Author: **Liz Langley** Target word: **Misconception**
2. Context Teacher contextualises the word within the text/activity	The article we are about to read is about a misconception
3. Repeat Students repeat the word	What's the word? Misconception

(continued)

(continued)

4. Friendly Definition Teacher provides a friendly definition of the word	A misconception is an idea that is not correct. You could also call it a myth
5. Teacher Examples Teacher provides examples in contexts other than the one in the text/activity	There are many fears and misconceptions about cancer I think people have the *misconception* that restaurants make a lot of money It is a misconception that you have to wait 24 h before filing a missing person report
6. Repeat Students repeat the word.	What's the word? misconception
7. Interaction Teacher creates a situation/activity where the students 'interact' with the word	I'm going to say some things and if you think they are a misconception that kids could have, say 'misconception'; if you think they are correct, say nothing – Chocolate milk comes from brown cows – The sky is blue – 1 + 1 = 2 – If you dig a really deep hole in the ground, you will get to China
8. Students' Examples Students provide some of their own examples	Do you think you have ever had a misconception? You could say, I had a misconception when I thought…
9. Repeat Teacher says friendly definition and students say the word again	What's the word that means you have an idea about something that turns out not to be correct? misconception

References

Al Otaiba, S., Gillespie Rouse, A., & Baker, K. (2018). Elementary grade intervention approaches to treat specific learning disabilities, including dyslexia. *Language, Speech, and Hearing Services in Schools, 49*(4), 829–842. https://doi.org/10.1044/2018_LSHSS-DYSLC-18-0022.

Allen, J. (1999). *Words, words, words: Teaching vocabulary in Grades 4-12.* Portland, ME: Stenhouse Publishers.

Beck, I. L., McKeown, M. G., & Kucan, L. (2008). *Solving problems in the teaching of literacy. Creating robust vocabulary: Frequently asked questions and extended examples.* New York, NY: Guilford Press.

Beck, I., McKeown, M., & Kucan, L. (2013). *Bringing words to life—Robust vocabulary instruction* (2nd ed.). New York: Guilford Press.

Castles, A., Coltheart, M., Larsen, L., Jones, P., Saunders, S., & McArthur, G. M. (2009). Assessing the basic components of reading: A revision of the Castles and Coltheart test with new norms (CC2). Retrieved from www.motif.org.au.

Clarke, P. J., Snowling, M. J., Truelove, E., & Hulme, C. (2010). Ameliorating children's reading-comprehension difficulties: A randomized controlled trial. *Psychological Science, 21*(8), 1106–1116.

Clarke, P. J., Truelove, E., Hulme, C., & Snowling, M. (2014). *Developing reading comprehension* (1st ed.). Hoboken: Wiley.

Cohen, J. (1988). *Statistical power analysis for the behavioral sciences* (2nd ed.). Hillsdale, NJ: Erlbaum.

Dale, E., & O'Rourke, J. (1986). *Vocabulary building: A process approach.* Columbus, OH: Zener-Bloser.

Dawson, N., & Ricketts, J. (2017). The role of semantic knowledge in learning to read exception words. *Perspectives of the ASHA Special Interest Groups, 2*(1), 95–104. https://doi.org/10.1044/persp2.SIG1.95.

Department of Education, Training and Employment. (2013). *Read It Again-FoundationQ!* Queensland, Australia: Queensland Department of Education, Training and Employment. https://earlychildhood.ehe.osu.edu/research/practice/read-it-again-prek/.

Gillon, G., & Dodd, B. (1995). The effects of training phonological, semantic, and syntactic processing skills in spoken language on reading ability. *Language, Speech, and Hearing Services in Schools, 26*(1), 58–68.

Gillon, G., McNeill, B., Scott, A., Denston, A., Wilson, L., Carson, K., et al. (2019). A better start to literacy learning: Findings from a teacher-implemented intervention in children's first year at school. *Reading and Writing.* https://doi.org/10.1007/s11145-018-9933-7.

Goddard, Y. L., Goddard, R. D., & Tschannen-Moran, M. (2007). A theoretical and empirical investigation of teacher collaboration for school improvement and student achievement in public elementary schools. *Teachers college record, 109*(4), 877–896.

Hiebert, E. H., & Kami, M. L. (Eds.). (2005). *Teaching and learning vocabulary: Bringing research to practice.* Mahway, NJ: Erlbaum.

Justice, L., & McGinty, A. (2010). *Read it again-PreK! A preschool curriculum supplement to promote language and literacy foundations.* Columbus, OH: Crane Center for Early Childhood Research and Policy. https://earlychildhood.ehe.osu.edu/research/practice/read-it-again-prek/.

Larsen, L., Kohnen, S., Nickels, L., & McArthur, G. (2015). The Letter-Sound Test (LeST): A reliable and valid comprehensive measure of grapheme–phoneme knowledge. *Australian Journal of Learning Difficulties, 20*(2), 129–142. https://doi.org/10.1080/19404158.2015.1037323.

Lathouras, M., Westerveld, M., & Trembath, D. (2019). Longitudinal reading outcomes in response to a book-based, whole class intervention for students from diverse cultural, linguistic and socio-economic backgrounds. *Australian Journal of Learning Difficulties, 24,* 147–161. https://doi.org/10.1080/19404158.2019.1640755.

Lennox, M., Westerveld, M. F., & Trembath, D. (2018). Evaluating the effectiveness of PrepSTART for promoting oral language and emergent literacy skills in disadvantaged preparatory students. *International Journal of Speech-Language Pathology, 20*(2), 191–201. https://doi.org/10.1080/17549507.2016.1229030.

Lindamood, P. C., & Lindamood, P. (2004). *Lindamood auditory conceptualization test: Examiner's manual.* Austin, TX: Pro-Ed.

Lindamood, P. D., & Lindamood, P. D. (2011). *Lindamood phoneme sequencing program for reading, spelling, and speech* (4th ed.). USA: Pro-Ed.

McGregor, K., & Duff, D. (2015). Promoting diverse and deep vocabulary development. In T. A. Ukrainetz (Ed.), *School-age language intervention: Evidence-based practices* (pp. 247–278). Austin, TX: Pro-Ed.

Milburn, T. F., Girolametto, L., Weitzman, E., & Greenberg, J. (2014). Enhancing preschool educators' ability to facilitate conversations during shared book reading. *Journal of Early Childhood Literacy, 14*(1), 105–140.

National Early Literacy Panel. (2008). *Developing early literacy: Report of the National Early Literacy Panel.* Washington, DC: National Institute for Literacy.

National Reading Panel. (2000). *Teaching children to read: An evidence-based assessment of the scientific research literature on reading and its implications for reading instruction* (Vol. NIH Publication No. 00-4769): Washington, DC: U.S. Government Printing Office.

Semel, E., Wiig, E. H., & Secord, W. A. (2006). *Clinical evaluation of language fundamentals—fourth edition—Australian* (4th ed.). Marrickville: Harcourt Assessment.

Snowling, M. J., Stothard, S. E., Clarke, P., Bowyer-Crane, C., Harrington, A., Truelove, E., & Hulme, C. (2012). *York assessment of reading for comprehension (YARC)*, (Australian ed.). London: GL Assessment.

Tomlinson, C. A. (2000). What is differentiated instruction. In Carolyn M. Callahan & H. L. Hertberg-Davis (Eds.), *Fundamentals of gifted education: Considering multiple perspectives* (pp. 287–300). New York, NY: Routledge.

Trivette, C. M., Simkus, A., Dunst, C. J., & Hamby, D. W. (2012). Repeated book reading and preschoolers' early literacy development. *Center for Early Literacy Learning, 5*(5), 1–13.

Wanzek, J., & Vaughn, S. (2007). Research-based implications from extensive early reading interventions. *School Psychology Review, 36*(4), 541–561.

Zucker, T. A., Cabell, S. Q., Justice, L. M., Pentimonti, J. M., & Kaderavek, J. N. (2013). The role of frequent, interactive prekindergarten shared reading in the longitudinal development of language and literacy skills. *Developmental Psychology, 49*(8), 1425–1439.

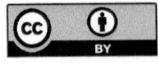

Chapter 6
Case Studies

Marleen F. Westerveld, Rebecca M. Armstrong, and Georgina M. Barton

Abstract In this chapter, we provide three case studies of students with different reading profiles. We demonstrate how using the five-step assessment to intervention approach explained in Chap. 2 assists in creating a detailed profile of each student's strengths and weaknesses in spoken and written language skills that are needed for successful reading comprehension. We highlight the importance of collaboration between professionals involved in the identification of students who experience difficulties in reading, to avoid duplication of assessments and to ensure targeted intervention can be provided by the most relevant professional at the required tier of intervention within a response-to-intervention (RtI) model.

Keywords Case studies · Speech-to-print profile · Reading difficulties

6.1   Case Study 1: James

James (S46: not his real name, age 9 years, 8 months) attended Year 4 at the school and had attended the school since Prep (foundation year). His enrolment form identified him speaking English as an additional language or dialect, but his teachers reported no concerns about his command of the English language. However, his teachers were concerned about his reading comprehension skills and had noticed difficulties in his spelling too (see Fig. 6.1). James' NAPLAN results (https://www.nap.edu.au/results-and-reports/how-to-interpret) were at the national minimum standard when he was tested in Year 3, particularly for writing and grammar and punctuation (reading band 3; writing band 2; spelling band 3; grammar and punctuation band 2). James performed at age level on the PROBE 2 (Parkin & Parkin, 2011); however, his performance on the PAT-R (Australian Council for Educational Research, 2018) was stanine 2, indicating performance well below expectations. When administering the *Reading Self-Concept Scale* (Chapman & Tunmer, 1995), James' response indicated average perceptions of difficulties, competence, and attitude. We investigated James' reading skills using our five-step assessment to intervention approach, as described in Chap. 2 (Fig. 2.2).

© The Author(s) 2020
M. F. Westerveld et al., *Reading Success in the Primary Years*,
https://doi.org/10.1007/978-981-15-3492-8_6

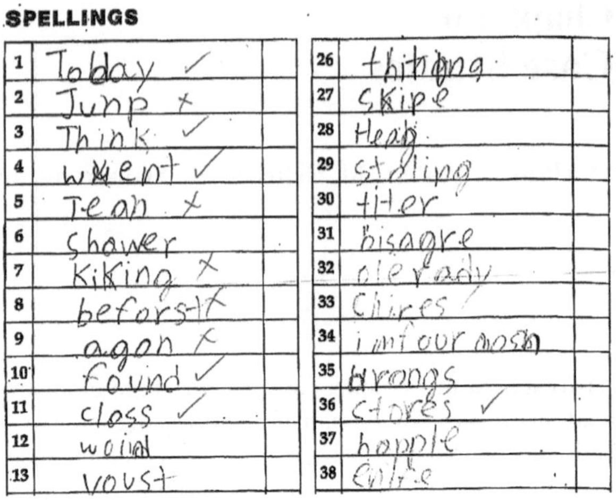

Fig. 6.1 James'
performance on the *Single
Word Spelling Test* (SWST;
Sacre & Masterson, 2000)

SPELLINGS

1	Today ✓			26	thithing
2	Jump ✗			27	skipe
3	Think ✓			28	Heab
4	wment ✓			29	stfling
5	Tean ✗			30	titler
6	shower			31	bisagre
7	kiking ✗			32	oleyady
8	beforslt			33	chires
9	agon ✗			34	imtour mosh
10	found ✓			35	Hyongs
11	closs ✓			36	ctores ✓
12	woial			37	bopple
13	voust			38	culire

6.1.1 Assessment Overview: Steps 1 to 4

Step 1: Assessment of Reading Skills

York Assessment of Reading for Comprehension (YARC; Snowling et al., 2012)
results indicated severe difficulties in reading comprehension (SS = 73; age
equivalent [AE] 6 years, 8 months).

Step 2i: Further Assessment of Students Who Scored Below Expectations: Check RA

James showed significant difficulties in reading accuracy (SS = 70, AE:
6;03 years), with 42.9% mispronunciations and 57.1% substitutions; and reading
rate (SS < 70; AE 6;0 years) on the YARC.

Step 2ii: Further Assessment of Students Who Scored Below Expectations: Check LC

James showed satisfactory performance (SS = 12) in language comprehension, using
the *Understanding Spoken Paragraphs* subtest from the CELF-4 (Semel, Wiig, &
Secord, 2006).

Step 3: Further Assessment of Students Who Scored Below Expectations on RA

Further assessment of word recognition, using the Castles and Coltheart test of single
word reading (CC2; Castles, Coltheart, Larsen, Jones, Saunders, & McArthur, 2009)
showed severe difficulties in single word reading across regular, irregular, and nonsense words (z's < −2.0). James performed poorly in orthographic knowledge (z =
−2.32 using Year 3 norms of the *Letter-Sound Test* (LeST; Larsen, Kohnen, Nickels,

& McArthur, 2015). Furthermore, James performed significantly below expectations (SS = 5) on the Elision subtest of the *Comprehensive Test of Phonological Processing* (CTOPP; Wagner, Torgesen, & Rashotte, 2013), indicating difficulties in phoneme awareness.

Step 4: Create a Speech-to-Print Profile

A speech-to-print profile was created based on the assessment results from Steps 1 to 3. The speech pathologist administered the *Rapid Automatic Naming* task of the CELF-4 which showed performance within normal limits. In addition, information was gathered from the classroom teacher, including James' performance on the *Single Word Spelling Test* (SWST; Sacre & Masterson, 2000) as shown in Fig. 6.1 (age equivalence 6 years, 9 months). James also participated in a curriculum-based assessment in English, based on the Novel *Rowan of Rin* by Emily Rodda. For this assessment, students had to explain how the author of this novel represents the main character in an important event. Students had to select an important event, complete several scaffolded tasks, including writing a draft, before producing a final copy of their response, which the teacher marked as not satisfactory for James' level of schooling (see Fig. 6.2). Because of the teacher's concerns about James' ability to answer some of the scaffolded questions and create a coherent response, the speech pathologist also administered an expository task (Heilmann & Malone, 2014) in which James was asked to explain his favourite game or sport. James chose to explain how to play soccer. The speech pathologist noticed James did not make effective use of the planning sheet in that he did not write down any keywords on page 1, but chose to draw a picture instead (Fig. 6.3). Although he used long sentences, he had difficulty formulating complex ideas and his explanation lacked cohesion (i.e. "*little discernible order to topics; much jumping between topics; and abrupt transitions between topics*"). The final speech-to-print profile is shown in Fig. 6.4.

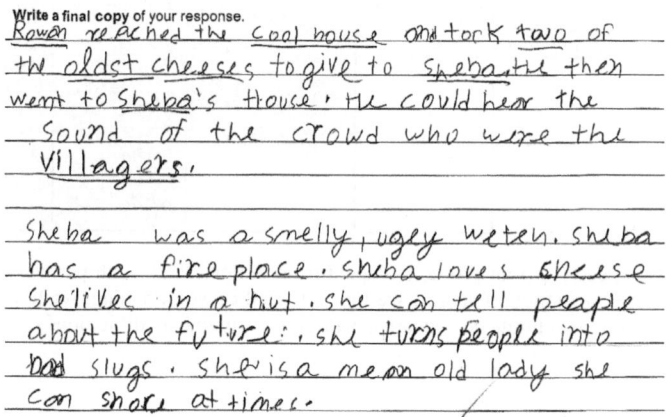

Fig. 6.2 James' final copy of his English assessment

Topic	What's Covered	Notes
What to Talk About When Explaining a Game or Sport		
Object	What you have to do to win	
Preparations	Playing Area and Setup Equipment and Materials What players do to get ready	
Start	How the contest begins, including who goes first	
Course of Play	What happens during a team or player's turn, including any special plays, positions, or roles, both offensive and defensive	
Rules	Major rules, including penalties for violations	
Scoring	Different ways to score, including point values	
Duration	How long the contest lasts, including how it ends and tie breaking procedures	
Strategies	What smart players do to win, both offensively and defensively	

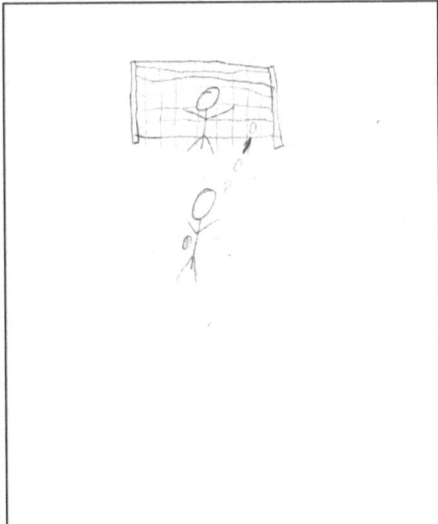

Fig. 6.3 James' expository planning sheet. (*Source* saltsoftware.com)

Spoken Language			Written Language		
Underlying representations	*Phonological Processing*				
Vocabulary knowledge	**Phonological Awareness**	**Storage and Retrieval**	**Rule/concept knowledge**	**Word – level**	**Text-level**
Syntax	*Syllable level*	*Non word repetition*	*Print concepts*	Word recognition	*Reading accuracy SS: <70*
Morphology	*Onset-rime level*	*Multisyllabic word repetition*	Grapheme-Phoneme Correspondences: *Z = -2.32 (Yr3 norms)*	*Regular word reading Z = -2.48*	*Reading comprehension SS: 73*
Phonology: No concerns	*Phoneme level Elision subtest SS: 5 (CTOPP)*	*Rapid Naming WNL*		*Irregular Z = -2.12*	*Reading fluency/rate SS: <70*
Text structure: Poor cohesion on expository generation task.				*Non-word Z = -2.62*	*Writing:* Teacher concerns – class example (Fig 6.2)
Understanding Spoken Paragraphs ScS:12				*Spelling:* teacher concerns (Fig 6.1).	

Fig. 6.4 James' speech-to-print profile (Adapted from Gillon, 2004, with permission from the author). *Note* for interpretation of scores, see Fig. 2.1 (Bell curve). Shading: white = not tested; light grey = within normal limits/no concerns; dark grey = significant difficulties

6.1.2 Case Discussion and Suggestions for Intervention (Step 5)

Based on the assessment results, it is clear that James has a profile of dyslexia (i.e. specific word recognition difficulties). James demonstrates reading comprehension difficulties due to his weaknesses in accurate and fluent word recognition skills, even though he shows adequate language comprehension skills. As explained in Chap. 1, these reading difficulties generally stem from phonological processing weaknesses; in James' case, he showed particular challenges with phoneme awareness tasks, but demonstrated age-appropriate performance in rapid automatic naming (i.e. phonological retrieval). James' difficulties in reading accuracy at sentence-level on the YARC were confirmed at word level on the CC-2, with significant difficulties on regular, irregular, and non-word reading. Moreover, James struggled on the LeST; closer inspection showed poor performance in naming of short vowels, digraphs, and diphthongs.

Worth mentioning is James' poor performance on the expository generation task, with limited use of complex sentences and poor cohesion. As shown in Fig. 6.3, James did not make efficient use of the planning sheet to organise his explanation of how to play the game/sport of his choice, soccer. James' difficulties on this task are most likely the result from reduced exposure to complex written materials due to his persistent word recognition difficulties (see also Chap. 1 for a discussion). Considering the emphasis on expository text from Year 4 of schooling (Snyder & Caccamise, 2010), this places James at high risk of facing challenges in most academic subjects, including English but also History and social studies.

Although James' teachers had been concerned about his reading skills, he had not been identified with specific word recognition difficulties. It seems likely that James' strong language comprehension skills masked his reading accuracy/word recognition difficulties during the early years of schooling. Early identification of James' significant difficulties in word recognition would have prompted early intervention. Considering the evidence that early intervention is critical for children with dyslexia to avoid long-term challenges in academic achievement and socio-emotional well-being, the importance of routinely use of sensitive reading assessment tools cannot be underestimated.

Step 5: Provision of Targeted Intervention

Based on James' profile (see also Fig. 6.4), he would benefit from intervention aimed at systematically improving: (1) his grapheme–phoneme knowledge; and (2) his phonological processing skills, making sure the intervention includes practice in spelling and reading to reach automaticity (see Al Otaiba, Gillespie Rouse, & Baker, 2018, for a review). Chapter 5 provides an example of an intensive intervention for students with a profile of specific word recognition difficulties. In addition, James would benefit from explicit instruction in how to use visual planners when evaluating and/or generating expository texts to guide not only his comprehension, but also his ability to generate these types of discourse genres.

6.1.3 Case Study 2: Hannah

Hannah (S02: not her real name) attended Year 4 when she became involved in the Reading Success project. Hannah (age 9 years, 10 months) spoke English as her first and only language and had attended the school since Prep (foundation year). Hannah had been referred to the speech pathologist because of concerns about her spoken language skills when she was in Prep but had not been verified with speech-language impairment (SLI). Hannah's teachers were still concerned about her oral language skills and had become increasingly concerned about her reading skills. Hannah's NAPLAN results were at the national minimum standard when she was tested in Year 3 for writing and spelling in particular (reading band 3; writing band 2; spelling band 2; grammar and punctuation band 3). Hannah's performance on the PAT-R was stanine 2 (5th percentile), indicating performance well below expectations. Hannah's PROBE-2 results were not available. When administering the *Reading Self-Concept Scale* (Chapman & Tunmer, 1995), Hannah's responses indicated very low self-ratings for reading difficulties and reading competence, but a high rating on reading attitude. We investigated Hannah's reading skills using our five-step assessment to intervention approach, as described in Chap. 2 (Fig. 2.2).

6.1.4 Assessment Overview: Steps 1 to 4

Step 1: Assessment of Reading Skills

York Assessment of Reading for Comprehension results indicated severe difficulties in reading comprehension (SS < 70; age equivalent [AE] 6 years, 0 months)

Step 2i: Further Assessment of Students Who Scored Below Expectations: Check RA

Hannah showed significant difficulties in reading accuracy (SS = 73, AE: 6;11 years)—with 29.2% mispronunciations, 62.5% substitutions, 4.2% additions, and 4.2% omissions; as well as reading rate (SS < 70; AE 6;07 years) on the YARC.

Step 2ii: Further Assessment of Students Who Scored Below Expectations: Check LC

Hannah demonstrated significant difficulties (SS = 5) in language comprehension, using the *Understanding Spoken Paragraphs* subtest from the CELF-4 (Semel et al., 2006).

Step 3: Further Assessment of Students Who Scored Below Expectations on RA

Further assessment of word recognition, using the CC-2 showed severe difficulties in single word reading across regular ($z = -2.31$), irregular ($z = -1.37$), and nonsense words ($z = -2.42$). Hannah also performed poorly in orthographic knowledge ($z = -1.9$ using Year 3 norms of the LeST). However, Hannah performed within typical limits on phonological awareness on the CTOPP, based on her scores on the elision and blending words subtests (composite score 88; 21st percentile).

Step 4: Create a Speech-to-Print Profile

Based on the assessment results from Steps 1 to 3, a speech-to-print profile was created. The speech pathologist administered additional subtests from the CTOPP and found Hannah to score within normal limits in rapid naming (Composite score 94; 35th percentile), but below expectations on tasks measuring phonological memory (Composite score 76; 5th percentile). To obtain a complete picture of Hannah's spoken language skills, the speech pathologist also administered the CELF-4. It was found that Hannah showed significant receptive and expressive spoken language difficulties (core language standard score 63; receptive language composite SS 70; expressive language composite SS 61).

To investigate Hannah's spoken language skills at text-level in a context that is relevant to her school environment, the speech pathologist administered the *Test of Narrative Language* (TNL; Gillam & Pearson, 2004) which assesses a child's oral narrative comprehension and production skills across three formats: (a) the child first listens to a script without pictures, then answers comprehension questions, before retelling the script; (b) the child first listens to a story based on a sequence of five pictures, then answers comprehension questions, before generating a story with five new pictures; and (c) the child listens to a fictional story while looking at a picture (dragon story), and asked comprehension questions related to that story, before generating a fictional story based on a different single picture (alien story). Hannah obtained standard scores of five for narrative comprehension and oral narration, which yielded an overall Narrative Language Ability Index of 70, indicating significant difficulties. Hannah's speech-to-print profile is shown in Fig. 6.5.

6.1.5   Case Discussion and Suggestions for Intervention (Step 5)

Based on the assessment results, it is clear that Hannah has a profile of mixed reading difficulties. In other words, her reading comprehension difficulties stem from significant weaknesses in word recognition and language comprehension. It is interesting to note that Hannah performed within normal limits on phoneme awareness. This may reflect the fact that she had received phonological awareness intervention from the speech pathologist in Year 2. It is not clear whether this intervention included activities aimed at improving Hannah's grapheme knowledge (i.e. letter-sound correspondences), particularly more complex ones. Further inspection of her LeST results showed a mastery of all 26 letters of the alphabet (except for /i/ and /x/), but difficulty with most digraphs (e.g. /ng/, /gn/, and /igh/) as well as diphthongs. It

Spoken Language			Written Language		
Underlying representations	*Phonological Processing*				
Vocabulary: Expressive ScS:4 Word Classes ScS: 5	**Phonological Awareness**	**Storage and Retrieval**	**Rule/concept knowledge**	**Word – level**	**Text-level**
Syntax Expressive ScS:3 Receptive ScS: 5	*Syllable level*	*Non word repetition SS:76 (CTOPP)*	*Print concepts*	Word recognition	*Reading accuracy SS: 73*
Morphology	*Onset-rime level*	*Multisyllabic word repetition*	Grapheme-Phoneme Correspondences:	*Regular word reading Z = -2.31*	*Reading comprehension SS < 70*
Phonology: No concerns	*Phoneme level SS:88 (CTOPP)*	*Rapid Naming CTOPP: WNL*	$Z = -1.90$ *(Yr3 norms)*	*Irregular Z = -1.37*	*Reading fluency/rate SS <70*
Text structure: TNL: SS70 Expressive SS:5 Receptive SS: 5				*Non-word Z = -2.42*	Writing
Understanding Spoken Paragraphs ScS:5				Spelling	

Fig. 6.5 Hannah's speech-to-print profile (Adapted from Gillon, 2004, with permission from the author). *Note* For interpretation of scores, see Fig. 2.1 (Bell curve). Shading: white = not tested; light grey = within normal limits/no concerns; dark grey = significant difficulties

is also not clear if this intervention specifically included spelling and reading tasks aimed at improving fluency (automaticity). It is of concern that Hannah showed a relatively low self-concept when we asked her questions regarding reading using the Self-Concept Scale (Chapman & Tunmer, 1995), indicating she found reading difficult and that she was not very good at it. In contrast, she scored higher when asked about her attitudes towards reading, highlighting she quite liked reading. As shown in Chap. 4, it is important to consider the students' self-perceptions when initiating intervention to ensure they are engaged in the process. In Hannah's case, a SWOT analysis would have provided invaluable information.

Considering Hannah demonstrated significant spoken language difficulties on standardised tests of language ability (the CELF-4 and the TNL), the speech pathologist transcribed Hannah's alien story (from the TNL), using Systematic Analysis of Language Transcripts, New Zealand/Australia version (SALT-NZ/AU; Miller, Gillon, & Westerveld, 2017) to perform a more detailed language sample analysis (Miller, Andriacchi, Nockerts, Westerveld, & Gillon, 2016). As shown in Fig. 6.6, Hannah's story was short, and showed a few grammatical errors, such as incorrect use of an article, referential pronoun, and noun-verb agreement. When comparing her performance to age-matched peers from the TNL database using SALT-NZ/AU, Hannah showed little use of complex sentences (low MLU: mean length of utterance); semantics (low semantic diversity in number of different words), and grammatical accuracy (in % utterances with errors). The SALT-NZ/AU database standard measures report is shown in Fig. 6.7 (with areas of difficulty highlighted in grey).

```
$ Child, Examiner
+ Language: English
+ ParticipantId: Hannah
+ Gender: F
+ CA: 9;6
+ Grade: 4
+ Context: Nar
+ Subgroup: TNL
+ Aliens
C there was a[ew] alien ship what[ew] just landed.
C and they were coming out.
C they were : a mum, a kid, a dog .
C and a dad.
C : and another girl.
C and there's a boy and a girl in the corner.
C and (the boy :02) the girl was trying to drag the boy.
C and the aliens[ew] girl : was waving.
C and the : girl : was shouting get the man to come out and say hello.
C and the little girl was leading the dog.
C and they looked like they were gonna Camp.
C that's it.
```

Fig. 6.6 Hannah's SALT transcript of the alien story (TNL, Gillam & Pearson, 2004). *Note* C = child; ew = error at word level; :02 = pause of 2 s

Next, the speech pathologist analysed Hannah's narrative at macrostructure level for the use of story grammar elements and cohesion (Hughes, McGillivray, & Schmidek, 1997). Hannah provided a description of the picture (i.e. characters), but there was little evidence of a problem-oriented narrative (i.e. problem "*and they were coming out*"), with no mention of a plan, actions, and a resolution. In Year 4, students are expected to produce true narratives containing all story grammar elements (characters, setting, initiating event, problem, plan, actions, resolution, and conclusion) across multiple episodes (Applebee, 1978). Considering the importance of narrative proficiency for classroom participation and academic achievement (Australian Curriculum Assessment and Reporting Authority [ACARA], 2012; Milosky, 1987), narrative intervention is clearly warranted.

Step 5: Provision of Targeted Intervention

Based on Hannah's profile (i.e. mixed reading difficulties), she would benefit from intervention targeting both her language comprehension and word recognition skills. Intervention for word recognition should aim to systematically improve: (1) her grapheme–phoneme knowledge; and (2) her phonological processing skills, making sure the intervention includes practice in spelling and reading to reach automaticity. Chapter 5 provides an example of an intensive intervention aimed at enhancing word recognition skills. In addition, Hannah would benefit from narrative intervention aimed at improving her story structure knowledge (i.e. story grammar) as well as her ability to use complex sentences (e.g. Gillam & Gillam, 2016; Westerveld & Gillon, 2008). Considering Hannah's significant reading difficulties, ongoing monitoring of her spoken and written language skills is clearly needed.

TNL Aliens coded

TRANSCRIPT INFORMATION	DATABASE INFORMATION
Speaker: Hannah (Child)	Database: TNL Narrative Samples
Sample Date: 4/8/2016	49 Samples Matched by Age
Current Age: 9;6, Grade: 4	Entire transcript
Context: Narration (TNL)	Context: Narration (Aliens)

STANDARD MEASURES REPORT

LANGUAGE MEASURE	Child		DATABASE				
	Score	+/-SD	Mean	Min	Max	SD	%SD
Compared to 49 Samples Matched by Age (ENTIRE TRANSCRIPT)							
Current Age (9;6)	9.50	0.22	9.43	9.00	10.00	0.33	3%
TRANSCRIPT LENGTH							
Total Utterances	12	-0.59	21.08	6	96	15.42	73%
# C&I Verbal Utts	12	-0.58	19.63	6	73	13.05	66%
All Words Including Mazes	86	-0.90	173.71	61	511	97.97	56%
Elapsed Time	---						
INTELLIGIBILITY							
% Intelligible Utterances	100%	0.28	98.99	76.92	100.00	3.62	4%
% Intelligible Words	100%	0.30	99.85	96.75	100.00	0.52	1%
SYNTAX/MORPHOLOGY							
# MLU in Words	7.00	-0.63	8.06	4.54	12.50	1.69	21%
# MLU in Morphemes	7.00 *	-1.03	8.88	4.92	13.43	1.83	21%
# Verbs/Utterance	1.25 *	-1.13	1.64	0.74	2.71	0.34	21%
SEMANTICS							
# Number Total Words (NTW)	84	-0.79	150.08	51	400	84.02	56%
# Number Different Words (NDW)	43 *	-1.15	73.96	32	140	26.85	36%
# Type Token Ratio (TTR)	0.51	-0.23	0.53	0.31	0.70	0.09	17%
# Moving-Average TTR (84)	0.51 *	-1.61	0.60	0.44	0.73	0.06	10%
VERBAL FACILITY							
Words per Minute	---						
Pauses Within Utterances	6 **	41.86	0.02	0	1	0.14	700%
Pauses Between Utterances	0	-0.14	0.02	0	1	0.14	700%
Pause Time as % of Total Time	---						
# Maze Words as % of Total Words	2.3% *	-1.24	10.59	1.20	27.67	6.65	63%
Abandoned Utterances	0	-0.52	0.41	0	3	0.79	193%
ERRORS							
# % Utterances with Errors	16.7% *	1.08	7.15	0.00	38.36	8.85	124%
Number of Omissions	0	-0.27	0.61	0	16	2.30	375%
Number of Error Codes	3	0.66	1.27	0	17	2.62	207%

Calculations based on C&I Verbal Utts
* At least 1 SD (** 2 SD) from the database mean
Moving-Average TTR based on a subset of 40 Database samples
Database selection criteria: age +/- 6 months (9;0 - 10;0)

Fig. 6.7   SALT—standard measures database report

6.2   Case Study 3: Bill

Bill (S38: not his real name) attended Year 1 of his local primary school. Bill (age 7 years, 1 month) had attended the school since the commencement of Prep (foundation year) the previous year. His enrolment form identified him as only speaking English in the home environment. At the end of Year 1, Bill demonstrated reading skills that were considered to be 'within expectations' for his Year level, with a PM Benchmark (Smith, Nelley, & Croft, 2009) level of 21 (with level 16 considered satisfactory at the end of Year 1). As part of the Reading Success project, we investigated Bill's reading skills using our five-step assessment to intervention approach, as described in Chap. 2 (Fig. 2.2).

6.2.1 Assessment Overview: Steps 1 to 4

Step 1: Assessment of Reading Skills

York Assessment of Reading for Comprehension results indicated severe difficulties in reading comprehension (SS < 70; age equivalent [AE] < 5 years).

Step 2i: Further Assessment of Students Who Scored Below Expectations: Check RA

On the YARC, Bill showed mild difficulties in reading accuracy (SS = 84, AE: 5; 10 years), with 14.3% mispronunciations, 71.4% substitutions, and 14.3% refusals. We were unable to calculate reading rate as the beginner level passage is not timed and Bill exceeded the maximum number of reading accuracy errors on Level 1 of the YARC.

Step 2ii: Further Assessment of Students Who Scored Below Expectations: Check LC

Bill showed language comprehension skills well below expectations (SS = 4), using the *Understanding Spoken Paragraphs* subtest from the CELF-5 (Wiig et al., 2017).

Step 3: Further Assessment of Students Who Scored Below Expectations on RA

Further assessment of word recognition, using the CC-2 showed difficulties in single word reading across regular (z-score $= -1.22$), and nonsense words (z-score $= -1.03$). However, Bill demonstrated satisfactory skills in irregular word reading ($z = -0.73$). Bill performed within expectations on the SPAT-R (Neilson, 2003); he showed difficulties in his orthographic knowledge on the LeST (z-score $= -1.04$).

Step 4: Create a Speech-to-Print Profile

A speech-to-print profile was created, based on the assessment results from Steps 1 to 3. The final speech-to-print profile is shown in Fig. 6.8.

6.2.2 Case Discussion and Suggestions for Intervention (Step 5)

Based on the assessment results, it is evident that Bill has a reading profile most consistent with mixed reading difficulties, that is, Bill demonstrated reading accuracy below expectations as well as difficulties with his language comprehension. In looking more closely at Bill's word recognition skills, it was evident that he had difficulties with his single word reading, including regular and nonsense words on the CC-2. He also showed poor orthographic knowledge. However, an area of strength

Spoken Language			Written Language		
Underlying representations	*Phonological Processing*				
Vocabulary knowledge	**Phonological Awareness**	**Storage and Retrieval**	**Rule/concept knowledge**	**Word – level**	**Text-level**
Syntax	*Syllable level SPAT-R WNL*	*Non word repetition*	*Print concepts*	Word recognition	*Reading accuracy SS: 84*
Morphology	*Onset-rime level SPAT-R WNL*	*Multisyllabic word repetition*	Grapheme-Phoneme Correspondences: Z = -1.04	*Regular word reading Z = -1.22*	*Reading comprehension SS: <70*
Phonology: No concerns	*Phoneme level SPAT-R WNL*	*Rapid Naming*		*Irregular Z = -0.73*	*Reading fluency/rate SS: Not calculated*
Text structure				*Non-word Z = -1.03*	*Writing*
Understanding Spoken Paragraphs SS: 4				*Spelling*	

Fig. 6.8 Bill's speech-to-print profile (Adapted from Gillon, 2004, with permission from the author). *Note* For interpretation of scores, see Fig. 2.1 (Bell curve). Shading: white = not tested; light grey = within normal limits/no concerns; dark grey = significant difficulties

for Bill included reading irregular words at the single word level, which reflects a strength in sight word reading. He also showed adequate phonological awareness skills when we administered the first seven subtests of the SPAT-R.

Bill would benefit from further assessment of his spoken language skills by the speech pathologist to determine whether his difficulties on the *Understanding Spoken Paragraphs* subtest of the CELF-5 stemmed from difficulties at word- and sentence-level. We would also want to check his ability to use spoken language at the discourse level, for example, to tell or retell a fictional narrative (see Chap. 2 for an overview of relevant assessment tasks). In addition, we would ask the teacher for classroom examples of Bill's written work, including the most recent results of a spelling test.

It is of concern that Bill's reading difficulties had not been identified by the school-based reading assessment, PM Benchmark. This assessment was administered at a similar point in the school year to the YARC. As outlined in Chap. 3, Bill is one of the 13 students (14% of the Year 1 cohort) who performed within typical limits on the PM Benchmark but showed significant difficulties on the YARC reading comprehension subtest.

Step 5: Provision of Targeted Intervention

Following the completion of the assessment, as part of the Reading Success project, Bill received access (without one-on-one support in a whole-class setting) to the Reading Doctor App by his classroom teacher to target his orthographic knowledge. Re-assessment on the LeST following this intervention indicated continued difficulties with orthographic knowledge (z-score = -1.62). Closer inspection of time spent on the app showed Bill was given access for only 56 min, reaching level 6 (out of 10). This is significantly less than the time spent by the students in Year 5 (see Chap. 5), indicating the importance of future research investigating the dosage effects of this type of intervention.

In terms of other support, Bill's narrative comprehension and production skills were assessed by the speech pathologist in Term 1, Year 2. He subsequently received small-group intervention targeting his narrative skills in Terms 2 and 3 of Year 2. These small groups were run by the speech pathologist at the school with support from a teacher aide. Following this intervention and on re-assessment with the YARC at the end of Year 2 (i.e. one year later), Bill demonstrated improvements in his reading accuracy (now SS 88) and reading comprehension (SS <70 to SS 86). Bill's reading rate continued to reflect difficulties (RR 76), though, suggesting he was still decoding at a slower rate than expected for his age. Considering the importance of fluent word recognition for reading comprehension, it is important Bill's reading skills are closely monitored.

6.3 Chapter Summary

In this chapter, we shared three case examples to demonstrate the usefulness of our five-step assessment to intervention framework (based on the Simple View of Reading) in: (a) determining which students may need further assessment of their spoken and/or written language skills, (b) understanding an individual student's strengths and weaknesses in the skills needed for successful reading comprehension, and (c) selecting specific targets for intervention. Both Year 4 students James and Hannah had performed at or above the benchmark on the NAPLAN in Year 3; both students showed difficulties on the PAT-R. However, further inspection revealed very different reading profiles, with significant implications for intervention and progress monitoring practices. Our case example Bill emphasised the importance of identification of reading difficulties during the early years of schooling and how timely intervention may assist early reading success. As outlined in Chap. 1, using the stepped assessment framework and its corresponding speech-to-print profile will thus encourage collaborative practice, by not only ensuring there is no double-up of assessments, but also by promoting a shared understanding between all professionals involved in the teaching of reading to aim for timely and effective instructional practices within a multitiered systems of support approach.

References

Al Otaiba, S., Gillespie Rouse, A., & Baker, K. (2018). Elementary grade intervention approaches to treat specific learning disabilities, including dyslexia. *Language, Speech, and Hearing Services in Schools, 49*(4), 829–842. https://doi.org/10.1044/2018_LSHSS-DYSLC-18-0022.

Applebee, A. (1978). *The child's concept of story*. Chicago: University of Chicago Press.

Australian Council for Educational Research. (2018). *Progressive achievement tests in reading (PAT-R)*. Australia: Author.

Australian Curriculum Assessment and Reporting Authority [ACARA]. (2012). The Australian Curriculum—English. Retrieved from www.australiancurriculum.edu.au.

Castles, A., Coltheart, M., Larsen, L., Jones, P., Saunders, S., & McArthur, G. M. (2009). Assessing the basic components of reading: A revision of the Castles and Coltheart test with new norms (CC2). Retrieved from www.motif.org.au.

Chapman, J. W., & Tunmer, W. E. (1995). Development of young children's reading self-concepts: An examination of emerging subcomponents and their relationship with reading achievement. *Journal of Educational Psychology, 87*(1), 154–167. https://doi.org/10.1037//0022-0663.87.1.154.

Gillam, S. L., & Gillam, R. B. (2016). Narrative discourse intervention for school-aged children with language impairment: Supporting knowledge in language and literacy. *Topics in Language Disorders, 36*(1), 20–34. https://doi.org/10.1097/TLD.0000000000000081.

Gillam, R. B., & Pearson, N. A. (2004). *Test of narrative language*. Austin, TX: Pro-ed.

Heilmann, J., & Malone, T. O. (2014). The rules of the game: Properties of a database of expository language samples. *Language, Speech, and Hearing Services in Schools, 45*(4), 277–290.

Hughes, D., McGillivray, L., & Schmidek, M. (1997). *Guide to narrative language: Procedures for assessment*. Eau Claire, WI: Thinking Publications.

Larsen, L., Kohnen, S., Nickels, L., & McArthur, G. (2015). The Letter-Sound Test (LeST): a reliable and valid comprehensive measure of grapheme–phoneme knowledge. *Australian Journal of Learning Difficulties, 20*(2), 129-142. https://doi.org/10.1080/19404158.2015.1037323.

Miller, J. F., Andriacchi, K., Nockerts, A., Westerveld, M., & Gillon, G. (2016). *Assessing language production using SALT software. A clinician's guide to language sample analysis. New Zealand—Australia version* (2nd ed.). Middleton, WI: SALT Software.

Miller, J. F., Gillon, G. T., & Westerveld, M. F. (2017). *Systematic analysis of language transcripts (SALT), New Zealand/Australia Version 18 [computer software]*. Madison, WI: SALT Software LLC.

Milosky, L. M. (1987). Narratives in the classroom. *Seminars in Speech and Language, 8*(4), 329–343.

Neilson, R. (2003). *Sutherland phonological awareness test - revised (SPAT-R)* (Revised ed.). Jamberoo, NSW: Author.

Parkin, C., & Parkin, C. (2011). *PROBE 2: Reading comprehension assessment*. Wellington, NZ: Triune Initiatives.

Sacre, L., & Masterson, J. (2000). *Single word spelling test (SWST)*. Windsor, Berkshire: NFER-Nelson.

Semel, E., Wiig, E. H., & Secord, W. A. (2006). *Clinical evaluation of language fundamentals—fourth edition—Australian* (4th ed.). Marrickville: Harcourt Assessment.

Smith, A., Nelley, E., & Croft, D. (2009). *PM benchmark reading assessment resources (AU/NZ)*. Melbourne: Cengage Learning Australia.

Snowling, M. J., Stothard, S. E., Clarke, P., Bowyer-Crane, C., Harrington, A., Truelove, E., & Hulme, C. (2012). *York assessment of reading for comprehension (YARC)*, (Australian ed.). London: GL Assessment.

Snyder, L., & Caccamise, D. (2010). Comprehension processes for expository text: Building meaning and making sense. In M. A. Nippold & C. M. Scott (Eds.), *Expository discourse in children, adolescents, and adults* (pp. 13–39). NY: Psychology Press.

Wagner, R. K., Torgesen, J. K., & Rashotte, C. A. (2013). *The comprehensive test of phonological processing—Second Edition (CTOPP-2)*. Austin, TX: Pro-ed.

Westerveld, M. F., & Gillon, G. T. (2008). Oral narrative intervention for children with mixed reading disability. *Child Language Teaching and Therapy, 24*(1), 31–54.

Wiig, E. H., Semel, E., & Secord, W. A. (2017). *Clinical evaluation of language fundamentals Australian and New Zealand* (5th ed.). Bloomington, MN: NCS Pearson.

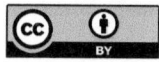

Part III
Findings from Teacher Interviews and Recommendations

Chapter 7
Feedback

Georgina M. Barton, Marleen F. Westerveld, and Rebecca M. Armstrong

Abstract In this chapter we share results from the qualitative data collected prior to (phase 1) and after completion (phase 2) of the Reading Success project. Information from staff interviews revealed some broader issues related to a whole-school approach to the teaching of reading. Findings showed several common themes, including the importance of positive and collaborative learning environments; having consistent language and communication across the whole school in relation to literacy education and more specifically the teaching of reading; and the inclusion of varied approaches that can be demonstrated for the purpose of professional learning.

Keywords Teacher interviews · Literacy education · Whole-school approaches

7.1 Phase 1 Staff Interviews

Initially, we were interested in knowing what the teachers and leaders thought about the literacy practices already being implemented in the school. We, therefore, carried out a number of interviews with staff involved in the teaching of reading at the school to find out what approaches and/or programmes were being used in the teaching of reading and whether the staff thought these were effective or not. It is important to note that these interviews were carried out at the beginning of the school's reform in literacy and reading instruction.

As outlined in Chap. 2, questions included: (1) What programmes are currently in place that aim to improve literacy (and more specifically reading) outcomes for students?; (2) What are the current perceptions of the success as well as areas in need of improvement of these programmes?; and (3) What future programmes and approaches to improving success in literacy learning might be considered in your school? We also gathered demographic information about the teachers that are displayed in Table 7.1.

Further, questions were semi-structured and focused on the approaches used within the school to improve literacy learning, and more specifically reading outcomes. Questions were based around the context of the school, the programmes being used for literacy, and what the teachers feel about the effectiveness of such

© The Author(s) 2020
M. F. Westerveld et al., *Reading Success in the Primary Years*,
https://doi.org/10.1007/978-981-15-3492-8_7

Table 7.1 Teachers' demographic information

Teacher pseudonym	Teaching experience in years	Current year level teaching	Qualifications
Lisa	4½	4/5	BEd—Early Childhood
Polly	15	4	BEd and Masters
Marie	4	4/5	Undergraduate and Graduate Diploma in Education
Geoff	15	Member of leadership team	Postgraduate Diploma in Education
Amelie	20	Not available	BEd Primary
Mina	30	5	BEd and Masters
Georgia	25	4	Diploma of Teaching

Note BEd Bachelor of Education

methods. We also asked what the teachers thought should be enhanced and how this could happen.

All interviews were transcribed and member checked (Koelsch, 2013; Oliver, Serovich, & Mason, 2005). The team all read the transcripts and wrote down any recurring codes and then themes (de Casterle, Gastmans, Bryon, & Denier, 2012). After initial themes were identified one team member took the lead on further analysis using an inductive thematic approach (Braun & Clarke, 2006) and consequently a number of themes were identified in these data including:

- The importance of a positive learning environment;
- A consistent language for literacy learning;
- Varied activities as well as a targeted approach;
- Cultural diversity.

7.1.1   The Importance of a Positive Learning Environment

All staff interviewed commented extremely positively about the school's culture and learning environment. They unanimously felt that the 'culture' of the school had been greatly improved over the past three years since the implementation of the Positive Behaviour Learning programme, called RISE. Having a consistent approach that was visible throughout the school via posters and slogans was making a difference. Staff believed that the students were willing to learn as a result and that parents were also aware of the school's overarching philosophy. This, in turn, had also impacted on the reputation of the school in the community.

> It's actually a really great school. The kids are really good. They're very positive. They love to learn which is great. You notice a huge change in their attitude towards school when they

hear RISE. So if you all of a sudden say what's RISE, they go, Respect, Independence, Safety, Effort and it's one of those things that's now drilled into them and they take it home with them which is really good too. There's a lot of visuals around the school which is great. It's a constant reminder for them. Lisa

Many of the teachers commented on how the school has a wide range of cultures represented in its school cohort. They felt that this diversity contributed to the positive learning environment established in the school. However, they also mentioned that a number of students come and go regularly which makes teaching them difficult. Overall, they felt the school had a good reputation in the community, which had not always been the case.

Probably low to mid socio-economic backgrounds, varied culture. Fairly, transient I think. Marie

I would suggest it is a school that is very multi-cultural but also very accepting. So we're a bit of a mixed bag. We've got high flyers, low flyers, different cultures all the way through. I actually think that it's a school that's really progressing forward. […] I think a lot of effort has gone into focusing on where the children have come from and then making them progress forward. Polly

7.1.2 A Consistent Language for Literacy Learning

All staff commented on a whole-school literacy approach that had been developed collaboratively over the past few years. The importance of a consistent language for literacy learning was highlighted by each interviewee. All staff believed that the six strategies for reading comprehension, for example, impacted positively on students' learning as it enabled teachers to focus on other areas of instruction; children were able to recite this quickly and move on to the next task. The reading and writing strategies, as well as differentiation and behaviour management plans as outlined in the school's improvement priorities (Table 7.2), were certainly having an effect.

The school recognised that professional development (PD) was an important component of all priority areas. Korthagen (2017) noted that both new and traditional approaches to PD are needed for teachers. He highlighted how a lot of "teacher learning takes place unconsciously and involves cognitive, emotional and motivational dimensions" (p. 387). Others have also revealed that professional development needs to be varied and not always top-down (Bahr, Dole, Bahr, Barton, & Davies, 2007; Hargreaves & Ainscow, 2015) and should take into account all teachers' needs. Bahr et al. (2007) offered a model of effective PD that notes the importance of teachers being able to choose the type of professional learning that suits their needs best. Further, the staff felt valued and that their voice was being heard.

In the last three years … new ideas coming out and they are monitored properly. Teachers are given time like this to sit down and discuss things and the peer observation we can go to other classes where teachers sit through what they're doing and then pick up something from there. Then they come to your class and they pick up something. There's a lot of opportunities. There's a lot of time factor given to us to collate all this information.

Table 7.2 The school's improvement priorities

Reading and writing	Differentiation	Behaviour management
Pedagogy	Pedagogy	Support
– Scheduled literacy blocks	– PD	– Positive Behaviour for
– Explicit teaching	– Coaching and mentoring	Learning (PBL)
– School reading framework	– Collaborative development of	– Internal PBL coach
– Jolly Phonics (Prep)	Individual Curriculum Plans	Strategies
– Robust Vocabulary	and Personal Learning Plans	– RISE
Instruction	– Evidence-based decisions	– Classroom rules
– Heggarty's phonemic	– Case management	– Behaviour matrix
awareness (Prep-2)	Support staff	– Official launch
– Read It Again	– Student support team	– STAR mascot
– FoundationQ! (Prep)	– Teacher aides	– STAR student of the
– Professional development	– Head of student learning	week
(PD)	– SEP teachers and aides	– Classroom behaviour
– Student goal setting	– Speech pathologist	walks
– Effective student feedback	– EAL/D teacher	– Time out buddies
– Running records	– Guidance officer	– Newsletter
– Moderation	– External agencies	PD
– Differentiation	Support programmes	– PBL tiers and
– Reading data wall	– Intervention programmes	visualisation
– Whole-school home	– Extension programmes, e.g.	– Effective behaviour
reading approach	robotics, U2B	management strategies
Support	– Social skills	– Behaviour data trends
– Master Teacher and Head	– Mindfulness—growth	
of Curriculum	coaching	
– Peer coaching		
– Student support team		
– Planning meetings		
– PD		
– Instructional feedback		
(five weeks)		

Generally, the staff felt supported in their work in the teaching of reading and noted that there were a number of improvements that had been happening over the past year, since the implementation of the school's reading plan.

> Our school's very focussed at the moment in terms of reading. Literacy is a really big push for us, especially reading. We do a lot of data meetings and collaborative meetings based around reading. We've got a huge data wall that we use to track how the kids are going in terms of the age appropriate level and their year level targets. We are just constantly focussing on reading and trying to improve it. Lisa

> A couple of years ago we developed a framework to try and have consistent language and consistent practices. It takes time to implement. It takes time to up-skill teachers and it takes time – that's continuous. But it takes time also to monitor it and to offer support and coaching, etc. Part of it was around consistent strategies in oral reading, as such and strategising comprehension. So there are two elements to it. Geoff

7.1.3 Varied Activities as well as a Targeted Approach

Another area mentioned consistently by staff was not only the targeted approach involving the six strategies but also the fact that their literacy plans consisted of varied activities for the students. Even though staff were asked to implement three literacy blocks per week that included guided reading activities, they were also able to develop and implement a range of pedagogical approaches to ensure all students' needs were met. Included in these activities were:

- Learning support lessons;
- Small group work;
- Explicit instruction;
- Time for reading;
- Guided reading;
- Comprehension skills;
- Text variance;
- Literacy blocks.

While the variety of activities was seen to be important, some staff did find there was limited flexibility due to time constraints and the requirement to do three literacy blocks each week. Further, some staff felt the need for more professional development on guided reading and that there were just too many expectations as to what to use in the classroom. Teachers still wanted more experience around particular teaching strategies in comprehension and in particular inferential comprehension.

7.1.4 Cultural Diversity

When staff described their school they were all well aware of the range of cultural diversity present in the student cohort—with 33% of students from ESL/EAL backgrounds and 6% Indigenous. While they mentioned this as a challenge, they also believed it was strength of the school. Interestingly, some of the staff were also from culturally diverse backgrounds and had extensive knowledge of different pedagogical approaches that supported diverse students' learning needs. Two staff members, for example, spoke about the importance of having a range of bilingual resources such as early readers in other languages for the children. They also recognised the need to acknowledge what the children bring to school with them from home in terms of experience. Similarly, some staff mentioned the need to improve the school's partnership with the community via a range of ways.

7.2   Phase 2 Staff Interviews

After the project was completed, a number of interviews with the staff who were available as arranged by the deputy principal, were conducted by an independent research assistant. Post-interviews involved Lisa, Polly, Marie, and Georgia. The same analytical process was carried out in this phase as in Phase 1, whereby codes were initially identified and then the codes were clustered into several themes. The themes in this phase of the project were identified as: communication, the importance of demonstration, a variety of strategies, and high expectations.

7.2.1   Communication

A strong theme from the second round of interviews was communication. All of the classroom teachers indicated that there was limited communication about the project's final results. They all felt that knowing the results of the children who participated in the intervention as well as how they improved would have been good.

> There wasn't a lot of communication…I didn't understand really in the end how… I guess if it was an improvement I would have liked to have seen the results. The post results for the kids that I had for those two years, because they are now in year six, and I've got no idea how they've progressed. (Lisa)

The teachers were also concerned about how the communication about the process itself was sometimes confusing. For example, Marie and Polly commented:

> I think one of the things that we had the most difficulty with to be honest was just the way that we were all communicating with each other about what was going on. (Marie)

> I don't really know anything else about the project … They were just being taken out to be tested with the speech pathologist in the last month or so… I know very little about it except that [it had] something that had to do with the university and that they were getting data and that sort of thing (Polly)

Additionally, the teachers indicated that they would have liked to know what the students were receiving in the small-group instruction. The teachers were, however, aware of whether or not they were a control group or not. They also knew about some of the measures such as the YARC, testing sound-letter correspondence, and the assessments that the speech pathologist was doing. Despite this, they all felt that knowing more about the results of the overall project as well as what activities the students were engaging in would have contributed to a more effective approach across the school.

> I think there was some improvement shown from the students that went, but for the rest of the class, I don't know that it had a huge impact. Like I said, we being the control group, we didn't really get much to support I guess. The kids were being taken out of the classroom to do it, so it was hard to know what skills they were being shown. (Georgia)

One of the positive aspects about communication about the project was that the teachers observed that there was now a consistent language being used across the school in relation to teaching of reading. This included the guided reading sessions as well as the robust vocabulary instruction. The teachers all felt these were both good approaches but more time reading and further understanding by the students about reading as a process would enhance the practice overall.

> Robust vocab is definitely a strength that we've got across the school. You talk about robust vocab to kids [and they] know exactly what you're talking about. Pretty much every class in the school have now got RVI walls. I think it just makes it come to the forefront of teachers' minds before they teach things. (Lisa)

7.2.2 The Importance of Demonstration and Professional Development

Another theme related to the second round of interviews was the importance of demonstrated practice. All of the teachers commented on how powerful it was for them to see someone else demonstrate and support their practice in the classroom context. This was particularly apparent with the Robust Vocabulary Instruction method. The teachers, however, would have liked to have seen a similar approach to some of the other activities related to the teaching of comprehension and decoding.

> And I think as a school we've just taken on some skills from the reading and we've actually applied it across the whole school level, so including smaller fluency groups, including smaller vocab groups, doing robust vocab in the whole school I think has really improved as well, so I think that's improved my skills, but also just a whole skill level. I thought it was really good because it was really good to be able to teach the robust vocab instruction and have someone set that example for us. (Marie)

Marie commented that having someone else show them what to do directly in the classroom with their students was extremely helpful. This also meant that the teachers were directly involved rather than, as previously explained, the students just being taken out of the class without the teachers knowing what activities they were doing. The teachers indicated that they would like more opportunities for someone to show them explicitly how to improve reading through a number of methods in their classroom spaces.

Another positive demonstrated practice was identified as the student SWOT interviews and speech-to-print profiles. The teachers agreed that these data sets told them specifically what the students needed once they were back in their mainstream classrooms.

> And I also thought it was really good that we had the interviews [and profiles] because we could actually see specifically what the kids needed in reading. It told us a bit more than just the general test, the diagnostic assessments that we would do with them in terms of PROBE and things like that. It actually broke it down into their phonemic ability and their phonological awareness, which was really good. (Marie)

The professional learning gained from direct experience was an important notion for the teachers and links with the theme of communication. It also aligns with the next theme of being able to utilise a range of strategies to improve reading outcomes.

7.2.3   Variety of Strategies for Teaching Reading

As per the first round of interviews, using a variety of strategies to improve reading results was encouraged by the staff. These strategies, it was also revealed, needed to be communicated and understood across the whole school. Teachers mentioned some of the consistent approaches that were expected to be implemented such as guided reading, robust vocabulary, and a number of comprehension strategies such as skimming, scanning, and summarising. The interviews revealed teachers were using a range of strategies, but they wanted to know more so they could support their students further:

> I think any focus on literacy, and vocabulary, and comprehension is a good thing. I think it did help staff across the school, because as a school we have actually adopted the specific instruction of robust vocab. It makes us think when we're doing whole unit planning, about the language involved, and the demands that are going to be needed from the kids to comprehend the task. (Lisa—second interview)

> We have a vocab group that we do when we're reading, and that's before they start to read. We've got a fluency group that we've got going. We obviously have independent and guided reading and things like that that we do. And then there's also a small group that comes up and admin actually works with them in terms of their phonemic awareness for those smaller groups, which is really good. And then as a whole class I do robust vocab for those texts that we do in the classroom, so it's really good. (Marie)

Despite the teachers having new knowledge about a variety of strategies, it was clear that more direct links between the classroom work and the Reading Success project were needed. As highlighted, a whole-school approach needs a comprehensive management plan that includes all methods being connected in meaningful ways. Unfortunately, both time and money were mentioned as inhibitors to such practices.

> We're looking at different strategies and we do reading groups and we've just started doing inferential questioning...We have a designated time when the children split into their differentiated groups reading and that's what I've been doing all year...They've all improved...I have six groups in my class and I have one group that go with one teacher aide for half an hour, and they're doing vocabulary and a cold read. After that they go to the fluency group the next day and in fluency group they are annotating the passage and after that they come to me and that's when I do the harder questions with them and we look at all the things that they've annotated and vocab that they don't know and then we do a really deep read and that rotates and keeps rotating. (Polly)

As described by Polly the teachers now have a bank of approaches they can use to support their students' reading progress. These, however, seemed not to relate clearly with the Reading Success programme.

7.2.4   *Having High Expectations and Celebrating Achievements*

An additional theme the teachers regularly mentioned was the importance of having high expectations and rigorous approaches to teaching reading. The teachers' discourse focused on how they were committed to supporting improvements in the students' overall learning and this required them to expect hard work and high achievement levels. They felt that the project did ensure that gains were made, particularly, for the students who may have been struggling more than others.

> Just to try, and lift the rigor that's in a guided reading lesson. And then the second program is, we actually have our leadership team coming in at least twice a term to actually watch, observe, and give specific feedback on our guided reading. The children know exactly what to expect from a guided reading lesson, and teachers are heavily supported in that process. (Lisa)
>
> And trying to find time and ways to do a more rigorous work, because in the half an hour, you can only do so much…I think it's more important that they're I guess having more time to look more deeply at the reading. (Georgia)

Finally, the staff believed that as the students were demonstrating improvements this needed to be reported to the whole school and community. Further, the leadership team acknowledged how teachers had learnt more about the teaching of reading and in particularly teaching vocabulary. Not sharing these successes could potentially make teachers and students feel their efforts are unrewarded. This sentiment also relates to the need for clearer communication of the results of the project generally.

7.3   Feedback from the School Leadership Team

When interviewing the leadership team, it became clear involvement in the Reading Success project had been a positive experience. When asked what the school had learned from their involvement in the project and whether it had changed the way they approached the teaching of reading, Geoff commented that:

> The Reading Success Project confirmed that our school is on the right track in terms of the targeted teaching of reading. It confirmed and highlighted the importance diagnosing individuals' needs and early and ongoing targeted intervention. It highlighted the fact that we need to invest more time into focusing on comprehension and as a result we have introduced 'Text Dependent Questioning' to help in this area.

The leadership team had appreciated the additional human and financial resources that were offered as part of the project which assisted the school in conducting the specific reading assessments and in providing the additional targeted reading interventions. However, there was acknowledgement of the need for ongoing professional development for teachers to help them accurately diagnose areas of needs and to develop specific teaching strategies to help make improvements.

However, the leadership team acknowledged the challenges faced during the project in *"finding a balance between the project's needs and the school's needs"*. Although Geoff said there were many positives to come out of being involved in the project, the school's main challenges in the implementing the model relates to time and resources:

> There is also a need to ensure teachers have the knowledge, skills and time to implement additional testing and to provide ongoing targeted teaching as a result of this. This requires a significant amount of time (ongoing) and resources. Developing a sustainable model is one of the challenges we face at a school level.

7.4 Chapter Summary

This chapter has shared findings from the staff interviews, prior to and following the school's involvement in the Reading Success project. Common themes within the staff interviews showed the importance of clear and consistent communication across the whole school in relation to approaches adopted towards teaching reading more generally, as well as the Reading Success project more specifically. The teachers, in particular, found demonstrated practice on a range of approaches to teaching reading extremely beneficial.

It became clear from the teacher interviews that communication regarding the specific results of the Reading Success project (both assessment and interventions) did not always filter back to all the teachers even though several professional development sessions were held with small teams of teachers involved in the project. Achieving whole-school reform is difficult, as acknowledged in the previous research (Fullan, 2007; McLaughlin & Talbert, 2006), particularly, in relation to literacy learning and the teaching of reading (Barton & McKay, 2016). Despite such challenges, it is important that all staff, students, and the community understand the particular approach being adopted and *why*. Chap. 8 will summarise what we have learned from the Reading Success project and how we may ensure these findings are shared with all stakeholders involved in ensuring reading success for all children.

References

Bahr, N., Dole, S., Bahr, M., Barton, G., & Davies, K. (2007). *Longitudinal evaluation of the effectiveness of professional development strategies*. Queensland: University of Queensland & Bond University.

Barton, G., & McKay, L. (2016). Conceptualising a literacy education model for junior secondary students: The spatial and reflective practices of an Australian school. *English in Australia, 51*(1), 37–45.

Braun, V., & Clarke, V. (2006). Using thematic analysis in psychology. *Qualitative Research in Psychology, 3*(2), 77–101. https://doi.org/10.1191/1478088706qp063oa.

de Casterle, B. D., Gastmans, C., Bryon, E., & Denier, Y. (2012). QUAGOL: A guide for qualitative data analysis. *International Journal of Nursing Studies, 49*(3), 360–371.

Fullan, M. (2007). *The new meaning of educational change* (4th ed.). London: Routledge.

Hargreaves, A., & Ainscow, M. (2015). The top and bottom of leadership and change. *Phi Delta Kappan, 97*(3), 42–48.

Koelsch, L. E. (2013). Reconceptualizing the member check interview. *International Journal of Qualitative Methods, 12*(1), 168–179.

Korthagen, F. (2017). Inconvenient truths about teacher learning: Towards professional development 3.0. *Teachers and Teaching, 23*(4), 387–405. https://doi.org/10.1080/13540602.2016.1211523.

McLaughlin, M. W., & Talbert, J. E. (2006). *Building school-based teacher learning communities: Professional strategies to improve student achievement* (Vol. 45). New York, NY: Teachers College Press.

Oliver, D. G., Serovich, J. M., & Mason, T. L. (2005). Constraints and opportunities with interview transcription: Towards reflection in qualitative research. *Social Forces, 84*(2), 1273–1289.

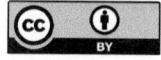

Chapter 8
Implications and Transferability to Other School Contexts

Marleen F. Westerveld, Rebecca M. Armstrong, Georgina M. Barton, and Jennifer Peach

Abstract This chapter starts by outlining what we have learned from the Reading Success project. Based on a summary of the main findings from the Reading Success project, we then consider ways in which the Reading Success project findings and practices shared in this book may be transferable to other contexts. We offer recommendations for best practice for schools wanting to investigate their current practices in the identification of, and support for, students experiencing difficulties in learning to read. We also describe some strategies that can be used by schools when striving for scalability. To finish, we provide recommendations on how the approach taken in this study might be adapted and adopted within other school contexts.

Keywords Scalability · Transferability · Educational implications

8.1 Introduction

It is undisputable that the teaching of reading is high stakes for all schools. Students' educational success relies on their ability to read fluently and to comprehend a range of complex texts. To implement the proposed interdisciplinary assessment and monitoring framework to assist in the identification of students experiencing difficulties in reading may require some schools to change their practice. Change is very much a constant in education, and it is important that these practices can be sustainable over time (Mioduser, Nachmias, Forkosh-Baruch, & Tubin, 2004). Pendergast, Main, Barton, Kanasa, Geelan, & Dowden (2015) discussed educational reform that targets improvement in student outcomes, and argued that educational change becomes increasingly more complex due to the different federal, state, and local systemic expectations. We understand that schools already have mandated literacy progress monitoring practices in place, such as NAPLAN at the federal level, and specific reading assessments at the regional level (see Chap. 2). One major challenge identified in the literature in relation to sustaining best practice is that schools are different to each other (i.e. no one size fits all) and that schools can rapidly change themselves. As suggested by Barton and Woolley (2017), to plan for change, the importance of an in-depth context analysis should not be underestimated (see also Thomson, 2010). In the next few sections, we will first provide an overview of

© The Author(s) 2020   141
M. F. Westerveld et al., *Reading Success in the Primary Years*,
https://doi.org/10.1007/978-981-15-3492-8_8

our take-home messages from the project, before briefly considering scalability and sustainability of our proposed framework.

8.2 Take-Home Messages From the Reading Success Project

The overall aim of the Reading Success project was to implement within the target school, a systematic process for identifying reading difficulties across the primary school years, using an evidence-based multidisciplinary approach. We believed that the introduction of an assessment and monitoring framework that was firmly based on the Simple View of Reading (Gough & Tunmer, 1986) would not only facilitate the early identification of reading difficulties, but would also enable timely and targeted intervention to address these challenges in reading. Moreover, creating speech-to-print profiles (see Table 1.2) for students who demonstrated challenges in reading served different purposes: (a) to highlight the underlying spoken language skills that are needed for written language (Gillon, 2018), (b) to encourage interdisciplinary collaborative practice in collecting assessment data, and (c) to ensure consistent language was used across the school.

The vision of the Department of Education is that every student in Queensland state schools receives the support they need to belong to the school community, engages purposefully in learning, and experiences academic and social success. Students experience inclusive education when they can access and fully participate in learning alongside their similar-aged peers, supported by reasonable adjustments and teaching strategies tailored to meet their individual needs. As highlighted in Chap. 7, it was clear that the school staff were highly committed to improving literacy learning outcomes for *all* students. It was evident that over the past three years or so the school had made great progress due to a number of strategies implemented around positive behaviour and reading. The school staff were extremely happy to be working at this school and commented on the nature of the school and students positively. This is of credit to all staff and the families at the school. Results from the interview data were overwhelmingly positive with also room for improvement.

The results from our project showed that the implementation of this assessment model was possible within a school context and successful in highlighting which students would benefit from more intensive reading interventions within a response-to-intervention framework (Fuchs & Fuchs, 2006). However, several issues came to light which may affect scalability, including time and resources, communication, and the need for professional development.

8.2.1 Time and Resources

Choice of Assessments

To meet the learning needs of all students, the Department has a commitment to a whole-school approach to quality teaching and improving student achievement. A whole-school approach directs support to different levels of need in response to student achievement data and is based on the premise that every student can learn and should have the opportunity to demonstrate progress on an ongoing basis. Implementation of a whole-school approach requires gathering and analysis of data that reflects departmental, regional, and school priorities and demonstrates the integral link between curriculum, interventions, and student outcomes.

At the differentiated level within a whole-school approach, cohort mapping provides the information teachers require to adequately differentiate reading instruction to meet the learning needs of all students within the curriculum. Teachers in schools have a range of cohort mapping tools available to them, such as Early Start for Prep—Year 2, and the National Literacy Learning Progression tool from Prep–Year 10 (www.australiancurriculum.edu.au) and it is up to the school team involved in the teaching of reading to decide which tools best suit their school's needs and are sensitive to early difficulties in reading performance. For young school-age students, these tools should relate to the development of the following six elements as discussed in Chap. 1 (see also Fig. 1.2): phonological awareness, phonics and phonemic awareness, oral language, fluency, vocabulary, and comprehension (Hempenstall, 2016; Konza, 2014).

To more accurately gather information about a student's learning rate and level of achievement, both individually and in comparison with a peer group, a combination of cohort mapping and progress monitoring is recommended. Progress monitoring ensures that all students, including high-achieving students are appropriately engaged, challenged, and extended, by designing class activities to meet students' learning needs, levels of readiness, interest, and motivation. Progress monitoring is used at a differentiated level to monitor response-to-intervention and may involve re-administering the cohort mapping tool or the use of curriculum-based measures. Progress monitoring is also used at focused and intensive levels but may be administered more frequently and will usually reflect the varying types of intervention individual students are receiving.

It became clear during the Reading Success Project that the school staff administered a wide range of assessments on a routine basis, for reporting, as well as progress monitoring purposes. Administering the *York Assessment of Reading for Comprehension* on a routine basis may be too time consuming. However, the results from this assessment greatly assisted in the early identification of students with different profiles of reading strengths and challenges. To determine if administering this specific test on a routine basis was needed within the school context, we conducted some comparisons with routinely used reading assessment tasks. Our results (Chap. 3) showed high correlations between student performance on the *PM Benchmark Reading Assessments* (Smith, Nelly, & Croft, 2009) and the YARC reading comprehension subtest during the early years of schooling, with excellent specificity and sensitivity data (i.e. > 80% of students were correctly identified). Our results also suggest that using a higher cut-off score on the PM Benchmark combined with a reading fluency task (e.g. TOWRE-2; Torgesen, Wagner, & Rashotte, 2012) may improve the sensitivity of this assessment.

A different picture emerged when comparing student performance on the *Progressive Achievement Tests in Reading* (PAT-R; Australian Council for Educational Research, 2018) to their performance on the YARC. About 20% of students were missed when using the PAT-R as a benchmark for reading competency, with these students showing very different reading profiles, despite adequate performance on the PAT-R. Therefore, use of the PAT-R on a routine basis may not only misidentify some students as competent readers, the results of the PAT-R will not help guide further assessment nor suggest which specific skills to address in intervention (see case studies in Chap. 6 for more information).

Taken together, our results show the importance of careful consideration of the routine assessments that are used to identify strengths and weaknesses in reading performance. As time is a precious resource, we recommend only administering high-quality assessments that are sensitive to ability and progress and will inform intervention.

A Team Approach to Differential Diagnosis

The importance of detailed diagnostic assessments to pinpoint individual students' strengths and weaknesses in reading comprehension is clear. It goes beyond the scope of this book to delve deeper into the potential underlying causal factors that may contribute to individual students' reading difficulties. While phonological processing deficits may be a primary cause of dyslexia or specific word recognition difficulties (see Table 1.2 speech-to-print profile), other cognitive skills such as attention and working memory may also play an important role (Catts, McIlbraith, Bridges, & Nielsen, 2017; see also Gray, Fox, Green, Alt, Hogan, Petscher, & Cowan, 2019). It is therefore important to carefully monitor progress in response-to-intervention and involve other members of the school-based interdisciplinary team (class teachers, speech pathologists, literacy support teachers, and guidance officers) in further assessment if students' progress is slower than expected. In some cases, an educational psychologist may be able to assist in providing a better understanding of each student's individual cognitive functioning, including their working memory profiles.

In summary, diagnostic assessments may be required to carefully describe individual students' strengths and weaknesses in reading comprehension in order to help target instruction and intervention appropriately. Differential diagnosis is time consuming and should only be used with those students who despite quality teaching and focused interventions are not meeting age- or year-level expectations. We recommend the use of increasingly diagnostic tools within a whole-school approach for students identified with reading difficulties, as per the process undertaken in the Reading Success project.

8.2.2 Communication

Positive outcomes of reform are possible if the whole school is committed to making a change in practice happen. In order to do this, effective and ongoing communication is necessary. As became clear in Chap. 7, the lack of direct communication between the research team and the teachers affected the teachers' feelings towards the project. During the course of the project, we mainly interacted with the leadership team through regular meetings, although several small-scale professional development and information-sharing events were held. Often in schools, leadership teams that include principals, deputy principals, and lead literacy or master teachers, make the decisions on what approaches to the teaching of reading are used in all classrooms. Known as a top-down model, this approach frequently results in teachers taking up mandated approaches rather than have a voice in change, with an increased chance of failure (Hargreaves & Ainscow, 2015).

Based on the teachers' feedback, we suggest that schools which consider adopting the evidence-based reading assessment and monitoring approach presented in this book develop a comprehensive communication plan across the whole school. This should include sharing and celebrating the results from projects, such as the Reading Success project, as well as other professional learning and development activities that have impacted positively on teachers' practices. In addition, we acknowledge the importance of taking a 'leading from the middle' approach (Hargreaves & Ainscow, 2015) that involves schools in an entire district, including the community. As Hargreaves and Ainscow argued when such an approach is taken schools will be better able: (1) to respond to local needs and diversities; (2) take collective responsibility for all students' and each other's success; (3) exercise initiative rather than implementing other people's initiatives; (4) integrate their own efforts with broad system priorities; and (5) establish transparency of participation and results (p. 44).

8.2.3 Professional Learning

One of the key elements in implementation of any new innovation is high-quality professional learning. This was an important theme that came out of the teachers' interviews (see Chap. 7). Graner and Deshler (2012) identified three key features of high-quality and effective professional learning. These are:

- Active participation of adult learners;
- Coaching, modelling, and instructional feedback; and
- Assessment of adult learning, implementation, and impact on student learning.

A large body of literature suggests that coaching, that is, individual teaching interactions between an experienced mentor and learner, enhances teachers' capacity to make changes in their practice, and that coaching within classrooms is a high yield strategy in delivering better literacy outcomes for students (see https://www.aitsl. edu.au/ for more information). Quality professional learning also has great potential to raise teachers' self-efficacy and sense of agency in relation to the teaching of literacy (Ryan & Barton, 2019). One way to support teachers' work in this area is to administer pre- and post-large-scale self-efficacy measures. (e.g. Tschannen-Moran & Johnson, 2011). In relation to the teaching of reading specifically, continued professional development as well as evidence-based approaches to supporting students' learning is needed. Given the highly politicised and public scrutiny of teachers' practices in classrooms greater support of, and trust in, teachers' professional judgment is recommended.

In the Reading Success project, coaching played a major role in the successful and sustainable implementation of Robust Vocabulary Instruction and Read It Again—*FoundationQ!* We suggest establishing an inclusive approach to mentoring or coaching in the classroom. Given each unique school context, it is advised the whole of staff discuss what this may look like but one approach would be to buddy up teachers with a partner and that time is allocated in the timetable for teachers to visit each other's classroom more regularly. These teachers then share their own practices with each other and then with another pair.

We recommend that all staff, including teaching staff, speech pathologists, teacher aides, and school leaders, engage in ongoing professional development on the teaching of reading within the Australian Curriculum. This professional development should consider diagnosis, support, and intervention at all levels within a whole-school approach with a focus on the 'big six' in reading instruction as outlined above. Further, whole-school professional development and training should be ongoing and involve a range of strategies such as intensive full-day professional development, formal and informal discussion amongst staff, coaching, demonstration, and inclusion of all stakeholders such as speech pathologists and other support staff.

It became clear from the teacher interviews that although a common language was used, not all reading practices were based on the most up to date evidence. For example, teachers' grouping practices play an important role in facilitating effective implementation of both reading instruction and inclusion of students with challenges in educational achievements. Flexible grouping allows students to move in and out of a variety of groups across learning areas and to benefit from collaboration with a wide range of peers. Flexible grouping is considered an effective practice for enhancing the knowledge and skills of students without the negative social consequences associated with more permanent groups (Tiernan, Casserly, & Maguire, 2018). With respect to reading skills, students can, for example, be grouped on the basis of interests and readiness, rather than ability. Research in inclusive education supports the practice of flexible grouping (e.g. Hanushek, Kain, Markman, & Rivkin, 2003; Justice, Logan, Lin, & Kaderavek 2014; Tiernan, Casserly, & Maguire, 2018). These studies consistently demonstrate that students' growth in various dimensions of achievement is influenced by the skill levels of their classmates, that these peer effects tend to be positive, and that these effects are largest amongst the least-skilled students.

8.3 Scalability

To promote adoption of the evidence-based interdisciplinary assessment framework described in this book, we now consider what steps are needed for transferability to a different setting. Scalability looks at whether a practice or an initiative can be implemented with similar or better results in other settings or with other groups. Scalability helps us understand when larger-scale implementation is appropriate and when it is not. Successful implementation of evidence-based interventions into education environments requires a systematic exploration of implementation strategies, to determine what works under what conditions. The following three strategies are important early in the process during initial implementation:

- Exploration strategies such as conducting a school-based needs analysis, determining stakeholder readiness or buy-in for innovation, and identifying specific barriers and facilitators of successful implementation.
- Education strategies to address material development and preparation, building educator capacity, professional learning, and methods of monitoring learning and performance.
- Financing strategies which focus on developing incentives to use innovations, providing support for professional learning and assessing the economic value of implementing an innovation (Fixsen, Blase, Naoom, & Wallace, 2009).

Additional strategies are needed when moving beyond the implementation in a single setting to multiple settings and may address staffing mix, professional roles, and physical and organisational structure to support innovation. A major challenge in scaling up new practices or models is to identify the policy that facilitates implementation of evidence-based practice, minimises barriers to implementation, and promotes the innovations at a state-wide or national level (Fixsen, Blase, Metz, & van Dyke, 2013).

8.4 Concluding Thoughts

In all classrooms, teachers are expected to provide differentiated instruction. Differentiated instruction involves active planning for student differences to ensure that every student is engaged and learning successfully (Tomlinson, Brimijoin, & Narvaez, 2008). Differentiated teaching means effective inclusion of all students in high-quality first teaching, scaffolding for all students, and standard adjustments that teachers can make to meet the learning needs of all students. As shown throughout this book, reading is a complex process and no two readers may demonstrate the same speech-to-print profile. Considering the importance of targeted intervention based on each student's reading profile, supporting students with reading difficulties in the classroom may thus be challenging. In our opinion, using an interdisciplinary and evidence-based approach to the timely identification of students at risk for or experiencing difficulties in reading at all stages of their reading development is a crucial first step when striving for reading success.

There are several key factors that enabled innovation and scalability in the Reading Success project. First of all, an education department with a strong commitment to evidence-based practice and an educational region that values and supports innovation and actively supports sharing of practice. Second, a leadership team in the school who recognised the integral link between spoken language and literacy and made the decision to allocate resources, both human and financial to ensure that all stakeholders were engaged and that programmes including Read It Again—*FoundationQ!* and Robust Vocabulary Instruction were delivered with fidelity. At the point of delivery, there were class teachers and speech pathologists who were open and brave enough to adopt an integrated service delivery model bringing together and enhancing the unique skills of each to create language-rich teaching and learning environments to support the educational outcomes for all students.

Although there are different philosophies around the teaching of reading, we worked collaboratively towards our common goal which was simple: *Reading Success* for all children. Ultimately, literacy is a basic human right.

References

Australian Council for Educational Research. (2018). *Progressive achievement tests in reading (PAT-R)*. Australia: Author.

Barton, G., & Woolley, G. (2017). *Developing literacy in the secondary classroom*. UK: Sage.

Catts, H. W., McIlraith, A., Bridges, M. S., & Nielsen, D. C. (2017). Viewing a phonological deficit within a multifactorial model of dyslexia. *Reading and Writing, 30,* 613–629. https://doi.org/10.1007/s11145-016-9692-2.

Fixsen, D., Blase, K., Metz, A., & Van Dyke, M. (2013). Statewide implementation of evidence based programs. *Exceptional Children, 79*(3), 213–230.

Fixsen, D. L., Blase, K. A., Naoom, S. F., & Wallace, F. (2009). Core implementation components. *Research on Social Work Practice, 19*(5), 531–540.

Fuchs, D., & Fuchs, L. S. (2006). Introduction to Response to Intervention: What, why, and how valid is it? *Reading Research Quarterly, 41*(1), 93–99. https://doi.org/10.1598/RRQ.41.1.4.

Gillon, G. T. (2018). *Phonological awareness: From research to practice* (2nd ed.). New York: The Guilford Press.

Gough, P. B., & Tunmer, W. E. (1986). Decoding, reading, and reading disability. *Remedial and Special Education, 7*(1), 6–10. https://doi.org/10.1177/074193258600700104.

Graner, P. S., & Deshler, D. D. (2012). Improving outcomes for adolescents with learning disabilities. In B. Wong & D. L. Butler (Eds.), *Learning about learning disabilities* (4th ed., pp. 299–323). US: Academic Press.

Gray, S., Fox, A. B., Green, S., Alt, M., Hogan, T. P., Petscher, Y., et al. (2019). Working memory profiles of children with dyslexia, developmental language disorder, or both. *Journal of Speech, Language, and Hearing Research, 62*(6), 1839–1858. https://doi.org/10.1044/2019_JSLHR-L-18-0148.

Hanushek, E. A., Kain, J. F., Markman, J. M., & Rivkin, S. G. (2003). Does peer ability affect student achievement? *Journal of Applied Psychometrics, 18,* 527–544.

Hargreaves, A., & Ainscow, M. (2015). The top and bottom of leadership and change. *Phi Delta Kappan, 97*(3), 42–48.

Hempenstall, K. (2016). *Read about it: Scientific evidence for effective teaching of reading CIS research report.* Australia: Centre for Independent Studies.

Justice, L. M., Logan, J. A., Lin, T. J., & Kaderavek, J. N. (2014). Peer effects in early childhood education: Testing the assumptions of special-education inclusion. *Psychological Science, 25*(9), 1722–1729.

Konza, D. (2014). Teaching reading: Why the Fab five should be the Big six. *Australian Journal of Teacher Education (Online), 39*(12), 153–169.

Mioduser, D., Nachmias, R., Forkosh-Baruch, A., & Tubin, D. (2004). Sustainability, scalability and transferability of ICT-based pedagogical innovations in Israeli schools. *Education, Communication & Information, 4*(1), 71–82.

Pendergast, D., Main, K., Barton, G., Kanasa, H., Geelan, D., & Dowden, T. (2015). The education change model as a vehicle for reform: Shifting year 7 and implementing junior secondary in Queensland. *Australian Journal of Middle Schooling, 15*(2), 4–18.

Ryan, M., & Barton, G. (2019). Literacy teachers as reflexive agents? Enablers and constraints. *The Australian Educational Researcher.* https://doi.org/10.1007/s13384-019-00349-9.

Smith, A., Nelley, E., & Croft, D. (2009). *PM benchmark reading assessment resources (AU/NZ).* Melbourne: Cengage Learning Australia.

Snowling, M. J., Stothard, S. E., Clarke, P., Bowyer-Crane, C., Harrington, A., Truelove, E., & Hulme, C. (2012). *York assessment of reading for comprehension (YARC),* (Australian ed.). London: GL Assessment.

Thomson, P. (2010). *Whole School Change: A literature review.* Newcastle upon Tyne, UK: Creativity, Culture and Education.

Tiernan, B., Casserly, A. M., & Maguire, G. (2018). Towards inclusive education: instructional practices to meet the needs of pupils with special educational needs in multi-grade settings. *International Journal of Inclusive Education, 1–21,* 01. https://doi.org/10.1080/13603116.2018.1483438.

Tomlinson, C., Brimijoin, K., & Narvaez, L. (2008). *The differentiated school: Making revolutionary changes in teaching and learning.* Alexandria, VA: ASCD.

Torgesen, J. K., Wagner, R. K., & Rashotte, C. A. (2012). *Test of word reading efficiency 2 (TOWRE-2).* Austin, TX: Pro-Ed.

Tschannen-Moran, M., & Johnson, D. (2011). Exploring literacy teachers' self-efficacy beliefs: Potential sources at play. *Teaching and Teacher Education, 27,* 751–761. https://doi.org/10.1016/j.tate.2010.12.005.

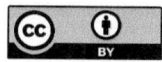